What I

Stop Being Stopped

"The health of our society is in crisis and people are desperately struggling to make lifestyle changes, The GO Doctor teaches us how to do it with passion, ease and grace"

—Mark Victor Hansen, Co-creator,
#1 New York Times best selling series *Chicken Soup for the Soul* ®,
Co-author, *Cracking the Millionaire Code* and
The One Minute Millionaire

＊　＊　＊

"The GO Doctor revisits what it means to be unstoppable and puts a unique twist on it. As a leading edge preventative medicine expert she opens up a whole new world of unstoppable health."

—Cynthia Kersey,
Best Selling Author of *Unstoppable & Unstoppable Women*

＊　＊　＊

"Working with The GO Doctor has turned the possibility of living a pain free, healthy and sexy life into a reality"

—Terri Levine, The Guru of Coaching SM,
President CoachInstitute.com and
Best Selling Author of Work Yourself Happy.

＊　＊　＊

"After reading the book I feel like I have spent my career in the dark and The Go Doctor has just switched on the light. I thank her for brightening my future."

—David Ford, World Champion, World Cup Champion,
4x Olympian and 2003 Canadian Male Athlete of the Year.

STOP BEING STOPPED

Uncle Lary & Auntie Sharon,

Thanks so much for your love, encouragment & support over all these years.

♡ Your neice,

Kn Paquette ND

"The GO Doctor"

STOP BEING STOPPED

The GO DOCTOR'S GUIDE to
Unleashing a Healthier, Sexier You!

Dr. Karen Lee Paquette, BS, BSPT, RCAMT, ND, CCC

iUniverse, Inc.
New York Lincoln Shanghai

Stop Being Stopped
The GO DOCTOR'S GUIDE to Unleashing a Healthier, Sexier You!

iUniverse books may be ordered through booksellers or by contacting:

iUniverse
2021 Pine Lake Road, Suite 100
Lincoln, NE 68512
www.iuniverse.com
1-800-Authors (1-800-288-4677)

Because of the dynamic nature of the Internet, any Web addresses or links contained in this book may have changed since publication and may no longer be valid.

The information, ideas, and suggestions in this book are not intended as a substitute for professional advice. Before following any suggestions contained in this book, you should consult your personal physician or mental health professional. Neither the author nor the publisher shall be liable or responsible for any loss or damage allegedly arising as a consequence of your use or application of any information or suggestions in this book.

ISBN: 978-0-595-42604-1 (pbk)
ISBN: 978-0-595-86932-9 (ebk)

Printed in the United States of America

In memory of my grandma, Emma Rohlen,
whose unwavering belief and investment
afforded me the opportunity
to follow my dreams
and turn them into reality.

Contents

Acknowledgments

I would like to extend my deepest gratitude to those individuals I have had the pleasure to encounter along my path to writing this book. You have all played a significant role in shaping my life and allowed me to touch yours. I would like to mention those who played a special role—without them, I could never have completed this book.

- My loving family, whose support and encouragement to follow my dreams allowed me to turn this book into a reality.

- My mother, Marion, for her love, knowing and investment in this project.

- My sister, Jodi, for lending her creative expertise in expressing beauty from the outside-in.

- My friend, Kempton Frederick, for sharing his unique ideas and providing the nourishment to complete this work through his exquisite culinary skills.

- My friend, Jonna Ebel, for giving me the gift of her intellect and experience.

- My friend Daniel Smachtenberger, for his generosity and guidance in shaping the overall content of this book.

- My internet and multi-media master, Keith McKenna, for providing more professional skills in one person than I could have hoped for in five and for his belief in our team.

- My publicist, Brigitte MacKenzie, for sharing her insight and enthusiasm, encouraging me to touch more lives.

- My angel, Mark Victor Hansen, for creating the title of this book and providing me with the knowledge and tools to turn my dreams into reality.

- My colleagues, Lyra Heller and Mike Katke, for permission to use their health questionnaire.

- My colleagues, Dr. Kristi Hughes and Lyra Heller, for graciously offering their consulting expertise.

- And, finally, iUniverse, for giving my book a physical presence and widespread public access.

Preface

In my profession as a physical therapist, naturopathic doctor, and life coach, I am often told of struggles, struggles of people desperately striving to look and feel their best. They not only share their struggles, but also tell of how failing, time and time again—to practice the principles of healthy living, such as eating a nutritious diet and getting regular exercise—has left them extremely unhappy with their appearance and overall state of health.

These same people ask me how I seem to do it with such ease. I tell them, quite simply, that I use the power of passion. When passion is the driving force behind your health, it's easy to integrate the principles of healthy living into your life.

So why do we struggle to integrate the principles of healthy living into our lives? Because we are being stopped, stopped by influences so strong that our efforts pale in comparison. Until we become aware of the detours and roadblocks that prevent us from tapping into our own unique passion for health, I guarantee you, we will continue to struggle, find only temporary results or perhaps fail completely. Knowledge of how easy it can be, coupled with my desire to help people ease their struggles, was the inspiration behind this book.

There are many resources that address certain aspects of a person's health, but addressing only part of a person's health is not enough. When I developed this material, I searched each of the four dimensions of human health—the body, mind, heart, and spirit—to find the one key element in each that is required to tap into our passion for health. This book shows you how to gain access to these four key elements, and when you incorporate these elements into your life, you just ooze sex appeal!

Imagine for a moment that you have found an unlimited amount of energy, an effortless sense of discipline, a tremendous power of will and, last but not least, an endless desire to nurture your health. Imagine waking up every morning with a passion so strong that you're excited to practice the principles of healthy living. What would your life be like then?

As you turn the page, you begin a journey of self-discovery that will forever change how you view your health. You will have the opportunity to complete The Fatigue Test, a health questionnaire that provides a unique window into your physical energy state. In addition, I have included "A Checklist for Staying on Course" to refer to as you encounter bumps on your road to looking and feeling your best.

If you would like additional assistance with creating your own personal road map to unleashing the healthier, sexier you, please refer to my Web site, http://stopbeingstopped.com, for continuing education specifically designed to pick up where this book leaves off. Starting right now, I give you the green light to begin the process that makes it easy to live life beautifully and healthfully for your very first time!

—Dr. Karen Lee Paquette, BS, BSPT, RCAMT, ND, CCC

Your Road Map

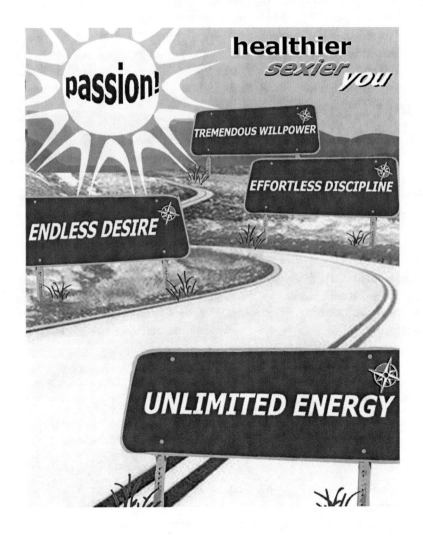

Let's Talk About Sexy!

Sexy as defined by Merriam-Webster's dictionary is "generally attractive or interesting: APPEALING and sexually suggestive or stimulating: EROTIC." Personally, I have noticed people using the word sexy in many different ways, and I would like to start by letting you know what I mean when I use the word.

When I think of the word sexy, I envision a person who radiates such an attractive and desirable energy that others are drawn in. It arrives most powerfully when we are living our personal best in all areas of our life, including our career, family and relationships. Living our personal best requires that we strive to optimize all four dimensions of our health: body, mind, heart, and spirit.

Sex appeal is not limited to a person's physical health and appearance; it encompasses much more than that. From the thoughts we think to the feelings we experience, from the spirit we radiate to our interactions with the world and everything that exists in it, it's all part of what makes up this powerful force called sex appeal. That's what I mean when I say "sexy," throughout the rest of the book.

After extensive clinical experience and investigation I have come to the understanding that the majority of people in our society do not feel sexy, at least as I describe it; rather they feel quite the opposite. My intention here is not only to provide them with an opportunity to redefine "sexy" for themselves, but also to move from wherever they are to wherever they desire to be.

Next, I will shift gears and lay some facts on the table. The facts confirm that the majority of people are desperately struggling to live life healthfully but are hovering in the space that I call the danger zone.

The statistics that follow are truly disturbing. I share them with you only to create an awareness of the truth about our culture's direction. It defines the point from which we look to the future, or as I like to call it, our *turning point*. I ask that you rally with me as we alter the course of our collective health and look toward a healthier, sexier future.

The Danger Zone

> *You can't determine which way the wind blows, but you can determine how you set your sails.*
>
> —*Anonymous*

Do you know that the number one cause of chronic disease is the failure to practice the principles of healthy living, such as eating a nutritious diet, getting regular exercise, and avoiding smoking?[1] As a result, conditions such as high blood pressure, elevated cholesterol, and obesity have contributed to a significant rise in chronic disease in recent years.[1] In fact, over 60 percent of adults in the United States[2] and Canada[3] are classified as overweight or obese.

Do you also know that seven out of ten Americans who die each year actually die of a chronic disease?[1] Heart disease, cancer, and stroke—all forms of chronic disease—have surfaced as the top three killers in the United States[4] and Canada.[5] What are these death and disease statistics telling us? Our failure to practice the principles of healthy living is, literally, killing us. And if we don't change our course, we are sure to arrive at destination—disaster.

So how are these devastating statistics affecting how we feel about our appearance? According to a recent *American Demographics* survey, when adults were asked to rank how happy they are with their physical appearance on a scale of one to ten, 47 percent gave themselves a score of five or lower.[6]

In another part of the survey, when women were asked about their quest for health and wellness, 87 percent said their quest for health and wellness motivates their life decisions more than anything else. In the same survey, 75 percent of women reported that they do not do as much for their health as they should, and 70 percent reported that they frequently do things that they know interfere with their well-being.[6]

It begs the question, if women's quest for health and wellness motivates their life decisions more than anything else, why are they not motivated to do as much for their health as they would like? Why do they frequently do things that interfere with their well-being? Why, when they have more health resources at their disposal than ever before, do they struggle to take care of their health?

Since I began practicing in 1994, people en route to destination disaster have arrived on my doorstep time and time again. What I've noticed, despite the diverse nature of my clientele, is that their routes are fraught with dangerous detours. Which detours they chose determined the nature of their struggle to integrate the principles of healthy living into their lives.

My intention here is to share these common detours with you so that you may become aware of which detours you take and how frequently you take them. This new found awareness will provide an opportunity to choose a new and more direct route to your destination—the healthier, sexier you!

The Detours

Detour # 1: Trading Health for Convenience

Our society, by and large, continues to chase the "American dream" in hopes of earning enough money to enjoy the possessions, experiences, and ultimately, the happiness we desire. To satisfy our desires, we dedicate a large portion of our time and energy to our careers, often at the expense of practicing the principles of healthy living, such as eating a nutritious diet and participating in regular exercise. The consequences of our choices are twofold, for failure to practice these principles both increases the stress we experience and denies us the stress reduction we would gain through practicing these principles.

When we choose to forego a nutritious meal in exchange for convenience foods, we are trading our health for convenience. When I use the term convenience foods, I mean calorie-rich, nutrient-poor foods. These foods are usually highly processed and laden with chemicals, artificial colors and flavors, additives, preservatives, and so on. Purchasing and consuming convenience foods on a regular basis not only increases the level of toxins in our body but also significantly reduces our intake of vitamins, minerals, enzymes, fiber, and balanced amounts of healthy proteins, fats, and carbohydrates.

The advent of convenience has had a detrimental affect on our activity levels as well as our diet. Technological devices such as automobiles, escalators, elevators, computers, remote controls, household appliances, and powered lawn mowers, just to name a few, all limit the amount of energy we expend. When time is at a premium, exercise commonly takes a back seat. Since we burn fewer calories, it is imperative that we intentionally build activity into our lives. I recommend that you make it a priority to eat foods packed with nutrition and to stay active, so that you don't trade your health for anything.

Detour # 2: Suboptimal Use of Health Care

Our current health care system excels in the treatment of urgent and emergent medical conditions. However, patients also tend to seek treatment from the conventional medical system for nonurgent conditions related to chronic diseases. When this type of nonurgent care is required, however, patients can also turn to the naturopathic medical system for guidance.

The naturopathic medical system excels in both the prevention and treatment of chronic disease brought on by failure to practice the principles of healthy living. Ideally, a qualified health care professional will help you find the root cause of your symptoms and provide you with the advice and education to restore and ultimately optimize your health.

When managing your health, seek and find out what is available within the realm of health care. Since both conventional and naturopathic styles have limitations, however, I advocate making the two work together to provide optimal care for you and your family.

Detour # 3: Our Mental-Emotional Programming

In our culture most of us learn to follow a mental and emotional map headed straight for disaster. Though our experiences are diverse, we have learned to see our appearance, thoughts, feelings, and actions as either good or bad, right or wrong, acceptable or unacceptable, or somewhere in between.

When we see things through the eyes of judgment, first we blame, then we feel shame, quickly followed by a dash of guilt. If that isn't punishment enough, we sprinkle a little more punishment right on top. When our actions are motivated by shame, guilt, and fear of punishment, they cannot be inspired actions. When are actions are not inspired from the inside-out, we are unable to tap into the power of passion. When we focus on judgment rather than on creating strategies that enhance our lives, we also diminish self-value, making it even more difficult to become passionate about our health.

> *When critical self-concepts prevent us from seeing the beauty in ourselves, we lose connection with the divine energy that is our source.*
>
> —*Marshall Rosenberg*

Detour # 4: Striving to Attain an Unrealistic Self-image

Since the advent of the mass media, we have been inundated with images of models, actresses and actors, TV personalities, and the rich and famous. With some genetic luck, hard work and dedication, makeup, extreme diet and lifestyle regimens, and sometimes a little plastic surgery, these celebrities have honed our idea of the perfect image.

In addition, technology now allows us to alter these images, so much so that the images are often no longer an accurate reflection of reality. It is these images that shape our perception and the perception of our children. It seems commonplace to compare ourselves with others and then begin a quest to match up to these images of perfection. More often than not, we subconsciously or even consciously judge ourselves as failures in this quest. When repeated, this destructive self-judgment degrades self-value and becomes a self-fulfilling prophecy.

Detour # 5: Subscribing to the "One Size Fits All" Mentality

As people, each of us is unique and deserves to be treated as an individual, especially when it pertains to our health. In pursuit of health and wellness, many of us reach out for help and are overwhelmed by the massive volume of resources.

Unfortunately, a large number of these resources claim that their recent scientific breakthrough, fad diet, or recycled lifestyle advice is the next miracle solution, and that, of course, it will work for everyone. This "one size fits all" mentality looks for quick fixes that produce only temporary results at best. The truth is that there is no single health solution for everyone. I advocate taking an individualized approach when it comes to managing and optimizing one of your most precious gifts, your health.

Detour # 6: Holding the "Quick-Fix" Expectation

Many of my clients have expressed the expectation that restoring and maintaining their health should come easily, without much investment on their part. They have simply not invested the time and energy, or maintained the patience required to achieve their health dreams. While some health concerns are mild and will resolve quite quickly, others require a long-term approach. To make lasting changes, I encourage you to consistently invest in your health.

I invite you to consider resetting your internal compass toward a new destination: the healthier, sexier you. To help you find your way, I have devised a road map that shows you where to avoid the dangerous detours and inefficient roadblocks on your road ahead. With your path clear and compass set, it's time to tap into the power of passion—the driving force behind your future success.

Passion—The Driving Force

Nothing great in the world has ever been accomplished without passion.
—*Georg Wilhelm Friedrich Hegel*

Why do some find it easy to practice the principles of healthy living while others struggle so? The answer, quite simply, is passion, passion, and more passion. Passion is the driving force inside us that overcomes all resistance. When you tap into the power of passion, it's easy to integrate the principles of healthy living into your life.

I would like you to picture yourself deeply immersed in the most passionate activity of your life. How does it make you feel? Notice how compelled you are to engage in it. No matter where your passion lies, be it in family, career, relationships, hobbies, or volunteer work, when you feel it, it energizes you. It is the driving force behind enlightened success. Tapping into the power of passion is something you already do in some areas of your life without even knowing it, and you can use it to turn your hopes and dreams into reality.

So how, you might ask, do we go about tapping into our passion for health? The answer lies in the four dimensions of human health: body, mind, heart, and spirit. In each dimension there is one key element that is required to tap into our passion for health. When all four key elements are effectively combined, previous struggles to live life healthfully just melt away.

What I notice about my clients who have a passion for their health is they have accessed the four key elements: an unlimited source of energy, an endless desire to nurture their health, an effortless sense of discipline, and finally, a tremendous power of will to say no whenever they wish.

What I notice about my clients who continue to struggle to live life healthfully is that they are stopped and do not have access to the four key elements required to tap into their passion for health. Taking down these roadblocks eliminates the struggle, providing an opportunity to design a personalized road map to take them from wherever they are to wherever they desire to be. This road map will take you there, too!

Seeing Your Stop Signs

> *So, once fairly on your way, don't stop because of some seemingly impass-*
> *able obstacle in front of you. What you want may be just beyond your nose,*
> *though you do not see it.*
>
> —*Thomas Edison*

I am sure that some of you are wondering how stop signs prevent you from achieving your health dreams. A stop sign is anything that stops you from accessing the energy, desire, discipline, and willpower necessary to nurture your health. Without access to these four key elements, you will be unable to use passion as the driving force to achieve your health dreams. The bottom line is this: if you don't become passionate about your health, you will always feel some level of struggle in nurturing it.

It's time to begin the journey through the four dimensions of your health to create your own personal road map. You will discover the most effective and efficient route to take on your road to looking and feeling your personal best. It will be devoid of both detours and stop signs. You will gain access to the unlimited energy to nurture your health, an endless desire to make your health a priority, the effortless discipline to act in accordance with your priorities, and such tremendous willpower that you no longer give into temptations that sabotage your goals.

I invite you to consider the ideas I present, try them on, see if they fit, and tailor them to your specific needs. My hope is that you will use the ideas to empower and inspire yourself to passionately and permanently integrate the principles of healthy living into your life. And finally, don't be surprised if you notice, as I did, benefits in all areas of your life.

Time for a Tune-up

Let's start by taking a close look at your physical health to determine if there are any stop signs that are preventing you from accessing unlimited amounts of energy, leaving you feeling fatigued and unmotivated.

For those of you who don't think that you suffer from a lack of energy, or feel your energy levels are adequate and are thus tempted to skip this section, I ask you to reconsider. Many of us mask our fatigue with the use of stimulants like coffee, tea, energy drinks, sodas, nicotine, and recreational drugs. These stimulants provide an energy boost that makes it difficult to determine our true energy levels. If you consume any of these stimulants, you may be masking a feeling of fatigue without even being aware of it. To find out, I recommend that you avoid consuming any stimulants for at least a week and monitor your energy levels. This will allow you to determine if you are using stimulants to avoid feeling fatigued.

In clinical practice, when I ask my clients to do this, only a handful report no significant drop in their energy levels. Prolonged use of stimulants stresses your body, eventually resulting in diminished energy levels and an even greater feeling of fatigue. Breaking out of this cycle is essential if you are to accurately assess your energy levels and optimize your health. Another factor to consider is the amount of stress you are under. People who experience high levels of stress secrete the stress hormone, adrenalin, which masks fatigue just as stimulants do.

No matter what their current level of energy, most of my clients say they could use a bit more. Just a few pages from now you will be asked to take The Fatigue Test, which will help you determine if your body is calling out for help. The results of this test narrow down the systems of your body that require attention and directs you to review personally relevant medical conditions. After reviewing the relevant medical conditions you will have a much better understanding of your overall health and you will be one step closer to finding out how fatigue may be affecting your life.

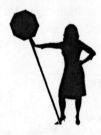

Destination I

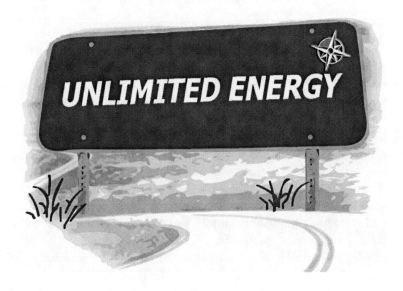

We are showered with information about living healthfully, but we have largely lost our sense of the body's wisdom.

—*Thomas Moore*

When I ask my clients what stops them from looking and feeling their best, the first of the most common stop signs I hear is, "I just simply don't have the energy." So what happened to their energy? Though stories and circumstances vary from person to person, the majority of people are responding to stress—chronic, low-grade stress. Currently, stress-related illness not only tops the charts for cause of death, it is also financially crippling, consuming a large portion of our governmental, insurance, and personal budgets each year in both the United States[7] and Canada.[8]

Part of my preparation for writing this book involved investigating stress-related illness and illnesses that list fatigue as a symptom. When I compared these lists, I realized that they were almost identical. One of the most common symptoms of a stress-related illness is lack of energy, otherwise know as fatigue. For the remainder of this book when I use the term fatigue, it is meant to encompass the feeling of being tired, lethargic, or not having optimal energy. When people experience fatigue, they find it very difficult to practice the principles of healthy living. As a result, fatigue is one of the most common stop signs we encounter.

Most people are not aware of how stress actually affects them. Some stressors are obvious, of course, but most are subtle, slowly wearing us out one day at a time. The cumulative effects of stress sneak up on us without our noticing, until one day signs and symptoms arrive. Stress affects the body in a series of physiological steps that I call the "stress cascade." This cascade is triggered when stress originates in any of the four dimensions of human health: the body, mind, heart, or spirit. This chapter focuses on the effect that stress, and its resultant fatigue, has on your physical health and what you can do to restore it. Subsequent chapters focus on to how to diminish the effects of stress in the other three dimensions of your health.

Physically, our bodies need to replenish whatever we deplete during the day in order to adapt to and diminish the impact that stress has on our health. It is simply a matter of addition and subtraction. For example, a nutrient-rich diet, regular exercise, and adequate sleep replenish our system. But small, seemingly harmless choices—not getting enough sleep, not eating the right food, not exercising, and turning to stimulants such as caffeine, alcohol, or drugs—deplete it. If we choose to deplete our systems more than we replenish them, even when our bodies seem to tolerate those depletions at the time, the body eventually hits a breaking point, and symptoms of stress-related illness, such as fatigue, appear.

Symptoms are your body's way of signaling that it can no longer adapt to stress on its own and needs help from you. First the body whispers, and if you don't hear it, it raises its voice, as symptoms become stronger and more numerous. If you continue to mute these signals, it will scream out loud with illnesses like diabetes, cancer, and heart disease. So instead of pushing the mute button, I encourage you to tune in to the whispers.

The Wear and Tear

The impact of stress on our health is an extremely complex cascade of events. I have simplified these complex interactions for you in hopes of providing you with a basic understanding of how stress directly impacts your health. I caution you: stress is a master of disguise, a chameleon. Each of the stress-related disorders associated with fatigue, marked in italics, is described in detail in the medical guide at the end of the book, titled "The Many Faces of Fatigue."

Please keep in mind that failure to practice the principles of healthy living, described later in this chapter, initiates the stress cascade and produces the same detrimental effects as mental, emotional, and spiritual stress. Here we go.

Sitting on top of your kidneys are two small glands, called the adrenal glands, that are primarily responsible for your body's reaction to stress. This reaction is designed to help you flourish under stressful situations by secreting stress hormones, one of which is well known, adrenalin. However, if the adrenal glands are more chronically overstimulated, they will respond by oversecreting cortisol, eventually leading to general adaptation syndrome, otherwise known as *adrenal dysfunction.*

Initially, under stress, it is cortisol's job to raise both your blood sugar and blood pressure. If stress is prolonged, persistent high blood pressure and *high blood sugar* can result. In response to high blood sugar, your pancreas releases a hormone called insulin. Insulin's job is to control sugar levels by moving the sugar out of your blood and into your cells, where much of it is stored as fat, directly contributing to poor body composition (too much fat relative to muscle), being overweight, and *obesity.* If your blood sugar remains chronically elevated due to continued stress or excessive sugar intake, insulin rises and can cause a sudden drop in blood sugar, resulting in *low blood sugar* levels.

If this situation is not resolved, your cells eventually become resistant to insulin, thus limiting sugar entry and failing to provide the cells with much-needed fuel to make your cellular energy, causing your blood sugar and insulin levels to rise. Chronically elevated blood sugar and resulting insulin insensitivity set the stage for acquiring type 2 diabetes. High levels of insulin signal your liver to produce cholesterol and diminish your capacity to break down fatty acids, resulting in elevated cholesterol and triglycerides.

Elevated insulin levels signal the body to lay down fat, otherwise known as belly fat specifically around the organs in your abdomen, contributing to abdominal *obesity* and *metabolic syndrome.* Belly fat releases substances known to contribute to *chronic inflammation,* damaging joints, blood vessels, and the immune system, and giving rise to conditions such as *fibromyalgia, coronary artery disease,* and *chronic fatigue syndrome.*

Inflammation, in turn, signals the adrenal glands to release more stress hormones, which trigger or worsen conditions such as *inflammatory bowel disease* and arthritis. By-products of inflammation known as free radicals contribute to *oxidative stress* and premature aging and increase your risk of acquiring chronic disease.

When you eat, your adrenal glands help regulate stomach-acid secretion. This acid breaks down your food so that it can be adequately digested, absorbed, transported, and assimilated into your body tissues. Initially, under periods of intense stress, stomach acid secretion can increase. However, prolonged, low-grade stress can lead to a decreased production of this acid.

As your partially digested food moves down the digestive tract, adequate stomach acid is needed to stimulate your gallbladder and pancreas to release bile and digestive enzymes. If stomach acid, bile, or pancreatic enzymes are inadequate, *maldigestion* of food occurs and either a generalized or specific *malabsorption* results. For example, essential fatty acid malabsorption contributes to the symptoms of *premenstrual syndrome,* and iron malabsorption contributes to iron deficiency *anemia.*

Adequate stomach acid has yet another role. It sterilizes the stomach contents and protects you from *small intestinal bowel overgrowth* and *yeast overgrowth.* In both of these conditions, the balance of microorganisms in your intestinal tract is disturbed and the digestive contents putrefy, producing gases, wastes, and toxins. This damages the integrity of your digestive tract and can result in *leaky gut syndrome.* A leaky gut allows inadequately digested food particles and toxins to enter the blood and lymph. Here your immune system recognizes them as foreign and launches an attack, better known as a food *allergy* and a milder form of immune response called food sensitivity.

When undigested food particles, disease-causing microorganisms, and their toxic waste products make their way through the digestive barrier to the liver, it is your liver's job to detoxify them. If it is overworked, a *sluggish liver* allows these substances to continue circulating in your system, thus polluting it.

Yet another role of cortisol is to regulate your immune system. With prolonged exposure to cortisol, your immune system can respond by becoming either under- or overactive. If an *underactive immune system* develops, it results in increased susceptibility to illnesses such as the common cold, flu, and even cancer. If, on the other hand, your immune system becomes too sensitive, it overreacts to environmental stimuli such as dust, mold, and pollen, in what are known as environmental *allergies.* This type of immune response can result in a change in the body's tissues, thus triggering the body to attack itself, manifesting as *autoimmune disorder.*

Eventually, stress hormones can inhibit the proper functioning of your thyroid, and it can become underactive. The thyroid gland is responsible for maintaining your temperature and your metabolic rate. An *underactive thyroid* makes it even more difficult to maintain a healthy body composition.

Cortisol, by depleting important substances in your brain, may also contribute to a decline in memory, mental fatigue, food cravings, *insomnia,* and a *depressed mood.*

As stress persists, your body can become depleted of the hormone DHEA, used by the body to make your sex hormones, and this in turn can inhibit your sex drive and contribute to *suboptimal menopause.* Finally, as the ability of the adrenal glands to churn out cortisol and other stress hormones declines, you move towards adrenal exhaustion, the final stage of general adaptation syndrome or *adrenal dysfunction.*

The stress-related conditions marked in italics above are all associated with a feeling of fatigue. This feeling of fatigue commonly arises once the ability of your cells to make energy has significantly diminished. What does this mean? It means that when you consistently feel fatigued, you are not only likely suffering from one of these stress- or fatigue-related medical conditions, but your cells are suffering right along with you. This cellular energy deficit is associated with a deficiency of the following nutrients: acetyl-L-carnitine, alpha lipoic acid, magnesium, vitamin E, coenzyme Q_{10}, and essential fatty acids.

More Wear and Tear

Our world is full of environmental toxins, including industrial pollutants, pesticides, automobile emissions, and heavy metals, just to name a few. These fatigue-generating chemical stressors significantly contribute to *environmental toxicity.*

Many of you undoubtedly take over-the-counter or prescription medications. Interestingly enough, fatigue is a common side effect of many medications, which makes it difficult to determine whether it is your medical condition or the medication that is responsible for your fatigue.

If you are taking any medication, prescription or over-the-counter, I strongly encourage you to read the list of possible side effects to see if fatigue, lethargy, listlessness, or any fatigue-like symptoms are listed.

Common fatigue-producing medications include antihistamines for allergies, antihypertensives to lower blood pressure, anti-inflammatories or corticosteroids to reduce inflammation, tranquilizers or sedatives used to induce sleep, and birth control pills to control the pain of menses and hormonal dysfunction as well as prevent pregnancy.

Many medications also deplete nutrients that are necessary for the maintenance of optimal energy levels. A qualified health care professional can help you identify and treat these depletions, potentially decrease the amount of medication required to manage your symptoms, or possibly eliminate the need for it altogether. If your medication has been prescribed by a medical doctor, you will need to work in conjunction with him or her if you wish to alter your medication regimen.

Regular Maintenance: The Principles of Healthy Living

Since failing to practice the principles of healthy living is the most common risk factor contributing to all chronic disease,[1] these principles can be used either to help resolve medical conditions that arise from chronic disease or to prevent it from finding its way into your life in the future. This list of healthy lifestyle habits will help you determine if poor dietary and lifestyle habits alone might be stopping you from accessing the unlimited amounts of energy required to look and feel your best. I can assure you that food, water, and lifestyle choices regarding sleep and exercise have a direct and immediate impact on your energy levels. How closely you adhere to these principles of healthy living influences both your general state of health and your risk of acquiring chronic disease.

Let's take a closer look at the Principles of Healthy Living that I have found to be most effective in improving health. These guidelines are principles to use to provide you with a basic foundation of health. To achieve optimal results I recommend that you create an individualized plan with a qualified health care professional.

Successfully and permanently integrating these principles of healthy living into your life will not only do wonders for your health, they will also reflect your sexy self!

The Principles of Healthy Living
Food Intake
Promote:

1. Eating frequent small meals, ideally five mini-meals a day.
2. Consuming food in a relaxed manner, chewing it extremely well before swallowing.

3. Consuming meals that consist primarily of fresh, organically grown, minimally processed green leafy and vibrantly colored vegetables, fruits, nuts, seeds, and legumes.

4. Consuming adequate portions of healthy protein at each meal including organically grown legumes, nuts, and seeds. If you choose to consume small portions of animal products, I recommend uncontaminated wild fish, wild game, or ethically and organically raised, grass fed free-range lean meats, eggs, and dairy.

5. Adequate intake of "good bacteria", healthy fats, vitamins, and minerals through dietary choices and, if required, intelligent supplementation.

Limit or completely avoid consuming:

1. Processed, canned, and packaged foods with additives, preservatives, artificial flavoring, and coloring.

2. Artificial sweeteners.

3. Fried and fast foods.

4. Foods high in refined carbohydrates, especially wheat flour and sugar.

5. Large quantities of animal products, especially those raised under unethical and unhealthy conditions.

6. The same foods over and over again with limited variety (this may create a sensitivity or allergy to them).

7. Foods that don't agree with you.

What you eat and how you eat it has an immediate effect on your energy levels. Failure to adhere to the suggestions above can contribute to the development of chronic disease.

Beverage Intake

Promote consumption of:

1. Plenty of chlorine-free, pure water each day. Your optimal daily water intake measured in ounces is one half of your weight measured in pounds. For example, if you weigh 150 pounds, it is recommended that you consume approximately 75 ounces of water daily.

2. Organically grown, caffeine-free herbal teas, high in antioxidants (If you choose to have a small amount of coffee or black tea, be sure that it's organic).

3. Large quantities of fluid away from meals, limit to 4 ounces with a meal (to prevent dilution of your stomach acid).

Limit or completely avoid consuming:

1. Large quantities of fluids just before bedtime so as not to interrupt your sleep.

2. Caffeinated beverages such as coffee, black tea, energy drinks, and sodas.

3. Beverages with added sugar, preservatives, or artificial flavor and color.

4. Alcoholic beverages.

Drinking suboptimal amounts of water, excess amounts of caffeinated beverages and alcohol has an immediate effect on your energy levels. Failure to adhere to the suggestions above can contribute to the development of chronic disease.

In clinical practice, once my clients have resolved any pertinent medical issues and are participating in a maintenance program, I suggest that they remain flexible with respect to food and beverage intake. This approach builds in freedom to enjoy meals out and be guests in other people's homes, and minimizes the stress that results from rigidity. However, it is optimal if the majority of their choices remain in line with the healthy habits I listed above.

Lifestyle Behaviors

Promote:

1. Regular exercise, being sure to include cardiovascular, resistance, and flexibility components.

2. Adequate and regular amounts of rest and relaxation.

3. Adequate and regular amounts of sleep (7-8.5 hours/night).

4. Use of environmentally friendly and chemical-free household and body care products.

Completely avoid or limit:

1. Smoking.

2. Use of recreational drugs.

3. Use of over-the-counter medications.

4. Exposure to toxic chemicals (e.g., pollution, substances in the occupational environment, household cleaning products, and body care products).

Sleep, exercise, and toxins have an immediate effect on your energy levels. Failure to adhere to the suggestions above can contribute to the development of chronic disease.

Some of my clients find reading the principles of healthy living educational in themselves, however, many of my clients arrive quite knowledgeable regarding the principles of healthy living and are looking for assistance in creating, implementing and monitoring an individualized healthy lifestyle program. If you would like my recommendation for a healthy lifestyle program please visit my website http://stopbeingstopped.com.

It has been my experience that as my client's energy level and overall feeling of wellbeing improve, the ease at which they are inclined to make healthy choices improves, naturally, right along with it. Integrating the principles of healthy living into your life not only reduces the stress that you experience but also provides a buffer for the stressors that you continue to experience. While important, these physical stressors are only part of health optimization. Utilizing effective strategies for preventing or defusing mental, emotional, and spiritual stress is equally important. These strategies are the focus of the remainder of this book.

Running Out of Gas

It's now time to turn to the Fatigue Test in "Your Medical Guide" at the end of the book and follow the directions for its use. Although lengthy, it is imperative that you complete the test in its entirety. Why, you might ask, have I not made the test shorter? Because I care about you, is the answer. All of my training and experience has taught me to be thorough, precise, detailed and holistic.

Each of your bodily systems is extremely complex. That's why we have medical specialists designated to assess and treat each one independently. However, they must all work together harmoniously to create optimal health. In this integrative questionnaire I offer you the opportunity to leave no stone unturned and start investing in you health right now. So please take as much time as you need to accurately complete the questionnaire in its entirety.

Once you have completed and scored the test, you will be asked to review the appropriate medical conditions listed in the section that follows the test, "The Many Faces of Fatigue." Please pay particular attention to the signs and symptoms listed under each condition, as they will help you determine which, if any, of the medical conditions discussed might be responsible for your face of fatigue.

Don't be alarmed if you experience signs and symptoms listed under many of the medical conditions. It does not mean that you suffer from them all. The signs and symptoms of fatigue and stress-related disorders show incredible overlap. The purpose of this section is to give you an idea about some of the most common physical manifestations of stress so you can begin resolving them.

At the bottom of each medical condition you will find some examples of the possible confirmatory tests you may choose to complete in order to confirm or rule out a particular medical condition. If you suspect that you may have found your face of fatigue and decide to work with a qualified health care professional, I recommend you bring your list to the appointment. Be aware, however, that some health care professionals will be more open than others to you taking such an active role in managing your health. You and your qualified health care professional will determine which, if any, tests are appropriate for your specific case.

The purpose of providing a list of possible confirmatory tests is to make you aware that there are objective assessment techniques and laboratory tests available to help you determine your face of fatigue. Once you have found your face of fatigue and take the steps to restore an unlimited sense of energy, you will be one key element closer to tapping into your passion for health.

Scheduling a Tune-up

If you scored *less than ten* in *all* sections of the test, congratulations! It is unlikely that a fatigue or stress-related medical condition is a limiting factor for you. You can implement the principles of healthy living discussed above as a general set of guidelines to live by. You may also explore a more detailed and individualized approach if so inclined.

If you scored *greater than ten* in any section of the test, reviewed the recommended medical conditions, and suspect that you may have one of them, I encourage you to make an appointment with a qualified health care professional to confirm your suspicions. Once a thorough assessment of your health has been made, you can begin the process of restoring your energy and ultimately your health.

If you scored *greater than ten* on *any* section of the test, reviewed the recommended medical conditions, and found no fatigue or stress-related conditions that apply to you, I still encourage you to make an appointment with a qualified health care professional. Remember, the test and medical conditions discussed in this book only provide an initial screening for common fatigue and stress-related medical conditions. There are many medical conditions beyond the scope of this book that you need to be screened for.

Appropriate health care practitioners include, but are not limited to, naturopathic doctors (designated as ND), functional medicine practitioners (includes MD, ND, DO, and DC designations), and naturally inclined or open-minded medical doctors. If you would like help in finding a qualified health care professional in your area, you can visit my Web site, http://stopbeingstopped.com.

You can evaluate the performance of your health care professional by how well they adhere to the following six naturopathic principles:

1. First and foremost, they *Do No Harm*. They use the gentlest methods at their disposal to facilitate recovery and optimize well-being, and when at all possible avoid use of substances that have devastating side effects.

2. After interviewing and examining you, they request or order any appropriate confirmatory tests, focusing on *Identifying the Underlying Cause* of your condition and co-create a plan with you that directly addresses your needs.

3. They devise a plan to *Treat the Whole Person*, with consideration of all four dimensions of your health, including the physical, mental, emotional, and spiritual. They look for and help you remove obstacles, which I call stop signs, that contribute to your struggle to optimize your health.

4. They monitor the valuable messages from the body, called signs and symptoms, and use methods that support the *Healing Power of Nature*. The healing power of nature refers to your body's innate ability to maintain and restore your health.

5. Their role of *Doctor as Teacher* is fulfilled by discussing, in terms you understand, the root cause of your symptoms, what factors (lifestyle and otherwise) are contributing to it, and suggest steps you can take to restore health.

6. Once your signs and symptoms have been alleviated and your condition resolved, the focus shifts to promoting *Wellness*. They guide you in nurturing your own health by continuing to teach you the principles

of healthy living and provide the support you require to optimize your health.

Next, and at the end of the following three chapters, I share my own personal story with you. My intention here is to show the information presented in this book in action, applied to real life. My hope is that you too are inspired to turn your dreams of health into reality.

My Road to Unlimited Energy

I remember a time when I was so tired that I didn't know how I was going to muster the energy to get out of bed in the morning, let alone prepare and consume nutritious meals, participate in a regular exercise regimen, and immerse myself in self-development as I once had.

In the summer following my third year of predentistry, I was involved in a car crash that altered the course of my career, and ultimately my life, forever. I had been the recipient of university scholarships in both volleyball and gymnastics. Following the accident, however, I was told by my team physician to cease all athletic activity and avoid exercise for the time being to let my body recover. But unfortunately it didn't.

I tried desperately to maintain my studies but found it extremely challenging due to the severe headaches and intense spinal pain that I was experiencing. I went from doctor to doctor, therapist to therapist in hopes of finding some relief, only to be met with a mountain of disappointment. The grim reality that I was never going to fulfill my career and athletic goals set in. In combination with lack of improvement in my physical health, my life as I knew it was over.

Several years later I experienced yet another tragedy. This time it was not initiated by physical injury; instead it was a mental, emotional, and spiritual blow to my health. I received a phone call informing me that my fifty-two-year-old father had dropped dead due to a sudden heart attack, with no warning. You can imagine my shock. In a split second I not only lost a parent, but also my mentor, my security, and my best friend.

That loss gave new meaning to the word pain, pain beyond what I could ever imagine. The physical pain and disappointment from the fallout of my car accident gained new perspective. It really didn't matter. Nothing mattered except that my father was dead and I would never ever see him again. There had been no warning, no preparation, and no chance to say good-bye.

The shock was like a drug and helped initially. I lived life in a trance, a robotic existence, interspersed with intense emotions and deep, deep sadness. Just when

I thought that life couldn't possibly get any more painful, the numbing trance started to wear off, little by little, allowing the pain to sink deeper, until every cell in my body was infused. As I struggled to get out of bed each day, I knew I needed to look inward to find the strength to move on, to continue the treadmill of life, and ultimately to find meaning in that struggle.

Eventually those tragic life events took their toll on me physically, mentally, emotionally, and spiritually. They left me suffering from chronic pain, fatigue, gradual weight gain, disappointment, sadness, anger, and ultimately a loss of love for life.

As I look back, I can identify many things that contributed to my lack of energy, including the fall out from the motor vehicle accident, the loss of my athletic scholarship and the opportunity to become a dentist, the death of my father, and my resultant poor state of health. Knowing I could not continue living my life as it stood, I dedicated myself to finding a more joyful way.

I was blessed to have found the medical expertise I needed to begin digging myself out of the hole I was living in. It provided me with the much-needed care I required. I received manual therapy, manipulation, acupuncture, energetic therapy, and prolotherapy (injections to stimulate the growth of ligaments and scar tissue), and I participated in a progressive exercise program to alleviate chronic pain, inflammation, and excess fat I had accumulated.

Once the pain and inflammation were under control, I focused on resolving the extreme fatigue that stopped me from fully integrating the principles of healthy living into my life. I began seeing a naturopathic doctor who helped me find my face of fatigue. Unfortunately, the traumas I had experienced initiated the stress cascade, and as the years passed, the effects of chronic low-grade stress took a toll on my health, and more specifically, my adrenal glands. I became aware that I was suffering from the effects of early adrenal exhaustion.

With my hopes high, I participated in a treatment plan that included dietary and lifestyle advice as well as taking the prescribed supplements, botanical, and homeopathic remedies to assist my own healing processes. I was elated when we had finally removed the first of my four stop signs, allowing me to regain access to an unlimited sense of energy.

My reclaimed energy provided the physical and mental stamina I needed to focus on restoring the next component of my health, my spirit. The force of the tragic blows I had experienced infiltrated my spirit, and I had lost my sense of desire to nurture my health. Attempting to discipline my mind and use willpower to overcome my struggles failed completely at this stage. I first needed to restore the desire to practice the principles of healthy living, for without that desire, it would be an uphill battle all the way.

To gain access to Unlimited Energy:

- Take steps to defuse your stress effectively by focusing your efforts on the dimension of your health where you believe the stress is rooted.

- Review the principles of healthy living and ask yourself, "Where can I improve with respect to living these principles?"

- Complete "The Fatigue Test."

- Review the medical conditions that apply to you, looking specifically for signs and symptoms that you experience.

- Take action to optimize your physical health by seeking appropriate treatment from a qualified health care professional for any signs, symptoms, or conditions that you suspect you have.

Destination II

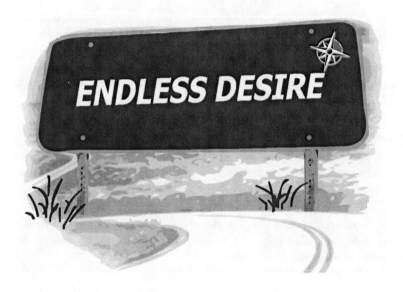

Champions aren't made in gyms. Champions are made from something they have deep inside them—a desire, a dream, a vision

—Muhammad Ali

When I ask my clients what stops them from looking and feeling their best, the second of the four most common stop signs I hear is, "I just don't seem to have the desire." The desire they are speaking of here is the desire to actually practice the principles of healthy living. It is important to note the difference between the desire to look and feel our best and the desire to invest the time and energy required to achieve those results.

Unfortunately, the vast majority of my clients desire the results and not the process. When I began working with clients in the mid 90s I noticed a common pattern. They arrived for their first visit, bright-eyed and bushy-tailed, with the desire to improve both their health and appearance. After an assessment we would design a plan that, if carried out, would certainly meet their goals. On follow-up, however, many would shamefully admit that they either partially or completely failed to carry out the plan. Others initially followed the plan but failed to adhere to a maintenance plan. What this experience taught me was that if my clients desired the process of carrying out the plan they would find it much easier to integrate it into their lives.

So where does the desire to nurture our health come from? It comes from recognizing the role our health plays in fulfilling our life's desire or our purpose—ultimately enhancing our lives and our world. When discussing this concept with my clients, I use the following analogy: Our bodies are the vehicles we use as we navigate our journey through life. How we care for that vehicle will in large part determine the destinations we can reach, the speed at which we can travel, and the comfort and joy we will experience along the way.

Just as our vehicles require fuel, new tires, regular maintenance, and upkeep, so do our bodies. Optimizing the performance and longevity of our transport vehicle through life requires that we embrace the principles of healthy living. If we fail to do this, we will find ourselves stranded at the side of the road, watching others pass us by in the vehicle of their dreams.

When I ask my clients to describe their life's desire, many admit that they have not consciously ventured there. Of the ones who have, only a handful are living, or at least working towards, that desire.

So how do we venture into the realm of desire? Desire is the emotion we feel when we envision the experiences we need or want to have when we interact with others and the world we live in. The greater the connection we make with our desires, the greater the access we have to an endless amount of desire to nurture our health. I discuss this idea in much more detail when we arrive at Destination IV: Tremendous Willpower, later in this book.

Our life's desire, however, is the feeling we experience when we envision fulfilling our life's purpose, ultimately enhancing our lives and our world. It is what inspires us to participate in life with vigor. In large part it supplies the energy to move in the direction we want to go.

Since the intensity with which we experience our feelings of desire is directly proportional to our connection to it, we need to first establish and then maintain that connection. When we connect with our life's desire we enhance our ability to act on that desire.

Our connection to our life's desire is found within ourselves, then enhanced in our relationships with others, with nature, and last but not least, our relationship with God or the universal energy at large. The more in tune we are with our life's desire, the more we recognize the integral role played by our health in carrying out that desire. So, to enhance our desire to nurture our health, we start by tuning into our life's desire.

> *When you are inspired… dormant forces, faculties, and talents become alive, and you discover yourself to be a greater person by far than you ever dreamed yourself to be.*
>
> —*Patanjali*

Designing Your Trip of Dreams

To enhance your sense of life's desire, you need to make a strong connection with your true self. Connecting with ourselves in our truest form is learning the essence of who we are at the depths of our being. When we hear what our true self is telling us, we begin to experience the feeling of desire associated with that truth.

Our true self is just us, in our most natural state. It is not who we think we should be or what others expect us to be. It's where our talents and gifts lie waiting to be unveiled to our friends, family, loved ones, and community. It's the little voice inside us that brings into awareness what we want, need and value. It knows us intimately, understands us completely and embraces all parts of our being.

It is only when we have a strong sense of our true selves that we can begin to tune into its wisdom. We can choose to either live in line with or ignore its wisdom. When we recognize and are inspired to use our unique talents and gifts, we have a sense of where we fit in and how we can contribute. When we are inspired to share our unique gifts and talents, we feel the desire to participate in life with vigor, a desire that is truly endless.

Sharing Your Trip of Dreams

When we unveil our true selves to our friends, family, lovers, communities, and the world at large by expressing our unique gifts, we create a deeper connection to our true selves and to our desires. The depth of connection depends on how authentic we are in expressing our true selves.

It's interesting how technological advances, on one hand, serve to enhance our connection to community and, on the other hand, serve to undermine that same connection. For example, access to mass media has improved our awareness of our global community but it can instill a sense of fear that limits when and where we go, whom we speak to, and how we behave. If we give into our fears and limit our depth of connection to our community, we experience feelings of isolation. When we isolate ourselves, it is much more difficult to feel connected to others, their unique gifts, and their desires.

This feeling of connectedness is a knowing that we are all brothers and sisters on this planet called Earth. It's a sense of compassion we feel for each other. We feel it with our children, families, friends and lovers. We even extend compassion to acquaintances and those we haven't even met. Compassion arises automatically when we hear a tragic story and want to reach out to help. This desire to reach out, in turn, deepens our feeling of connectedness.

When we use our unique gifts to contribute to the community and when we work together with others on projects near and dear to our hearts, our desire to fulfill our life's desire is magnified.

I would like to share with you an analogy that solidified this concept for me. When two people work together in connectedness, the outcome is not the result of basic addition, as shown in the equation, $1 + 1 = 2$. Rather, from a perspective of connectedness, 1 and 1 stand side by side and together become 11.

When we connect with the desires of others in our community and contribute to that community by following the desires of our truest self, it in turn feeds our own sense of desire. Recognizing the integral role that our health plays in the quality of life we lead, especially when we choose to fulfill our life's desire, is what inspires us to nurture one of our most precious gifts, our health.

Travel Insurance

The sense of desire we feel when we connect with our true selves and the community at large needs protection to ensure that we don't allow people we encounter and the challenges we face to dampen them. What I have found to be most effective in protecting our most precious desires when connecting with community is to carefully choose the people with whom we interact and how intimate those interactions are.

On a broader scale, protecting our most precious desires also requires that we maintain faith in our journey as we navigate through life. To keep our desires intact, we can use both our circle of influence and our faith.

Our Circle of Influence

I define our circle of influence as those individuals who have a direct influence on our lives. Since the people around us can influence our level of energy and the way we think and feel, it is wise to carefully choose where we place people in that circle. We protect our desires when we surround ourselves with people whose common goal is to coordinate their knowledge, effort, and intentions to enhance the lives of those involved and the world at large.

Choosing our circle of influence wisely requires that we first learn to recognize the people who clearly enhance or diminish our desires. It's easy to identify those who fit into these two extremes, but people whose toxic influence is more subtle somehow manage to fly under the radar and often remain unidentified. Without our being aware of it, time spent with these individuals can dampen our desires. With each interaction we improve our awareness of the effect these individuals have on our spirit. Once identified, we can manage our interactions with them more effectively.

What I have found to be most effective in helping my clients manage their circle of influence is a visualizing technique. I would like you to visualize a series of rings, one encompassing the next like layers of an onion. The nucleus or innermost layer represents you. The first ring surrounding you is your inner circle. It is reserved for those who have a significant and direct positive influence on your life and you on theirs. Next is a series of rings surrounding your inner circle. As you interact with people, place each individual in the appropriate ring, just the right distance from you. The distance is optimal for both parties, taking all factors into account. This allows you to maintain a relationship with all people at all times.

As time passes, individuals may remain where you initially place them, or they may move closer or farther away. Monitoring your circle of influence allows you to accommodate the natural ebb and flow of relationships in a harmonious fashion, without discarding anyone from your life.

Our Faith

Faith is the belief or trust we feel when we make decisions not solely based on logic or evidence. I describe faith to my clients as trust in the wisdom of the universe, or if you prefer, trust in the wisdom of God. When we trust that the universe is wise, that it knows precisely what experiences we require for our own personal development, we can maintain faith that the challenges we encounter have purpose. We feel, at all times, that we are exactly where we need to be to learn our valuable lessons. Our alternative is to resist. Keep in mind that resistance to what is creates stress, and stress acts to deplete our sense of desire to live life to the fullest.

If we maintain faith in the midst of our challenges, we are able to see them as having purpose and as part of a bigger picture. When we trust that our challenges serve a purpose, we find that we can experience the richness of life even within chaos. I encourage you to consider challenges as lessons and strive to work through them, rather than resist them. I invite you to see yourself as a student in the university called life and take the opportunity to learn from it. Adopting this philosophy gives us confidence to take risks, which is essential if we are to embrace personal development.

As we reflect on our challenges and celebrate as we move through those challenges, we gain strength. A strength that we couldn't previously have imagined we had. There is a strength within, triggered by crisis, that brings us a newfound perspective we wouldn't otherwise have gained. When we trust in the wisdom of the universe, we can maintain, protect and even fuel our desires by seeing our challenges as opportunities.

If we are unable to embrace our challenges in each moment, we can, upon reflection, return to faith. The knowing that all of our experiences, both pleasant and unpleasant, have a higher purpose. People, no matter how annoying or despicable they may seem, are in your life for a reason. Look upon them as teachers in this school of life. I ask that you strive to learn your lessons quickly and move individuals that do not enhance your life to your outer circle, ensuring that they do not dampen your desire to participate in life with vigor.

Our lives can at times be filled with trauma and tragedy. My intention here is not to minimize those experiences. I do not expect that you welcome cruelty. I present the concept of faith to encourage you to find peace after tragedy. Remember, the universe doesn't always hand us what we want, but it may hand us what we need. So set your sails in the direction you want to go and trust the wind to take you there.

My Road to Endless Desire

Following the cascade of events in my life that I shared with you in the last chapter, I realized that my career goals and my athletic and personal aspirations were never going to happen as I had hoped. As I struggled to get out of bed each day, I realized that I was up against a second stop sign, lack of desire. I had not only lost my desire to practice the principles of healthy living, but more importantly, I had lost the connection to my life's desire, the desire to live my purpose and enhance my life, the lives of those around me, and the world at large.

I began looking deep inside to find something I could grab onto to pull myself out of the dark cloud of doom that seemed to take hold of my spirit. I wanted so desperately to restore a sense of desire in my life, trusting that my desire to practice the principles would not be far behind. I felt completely alone and disconnected from the rest of the world because I thought that no one could understand my pain.

I focused my attention inward, looking to reconnect with my true self. The self I knew, the one who had something to share with the world, was deep inside. Improving my self-awareness, I connected with my true self through self-reflection, combining techniques such as deep breathing and meditation. I searched to identify my unique talents and how I could best contribute to my community by using those talents. I reveled in the beauty of nature, spending time outdoors, and connecting with mother earth.

Once I felt a strong connection to my true self, it was easy to see my calling. I was to help others by sharing my story and in turn listening to theirs. And so I decided I would spend time with my clients helping them resolve their physical pain and return to a fully functioning life. I knew that somehow, through my connection to community, I would be able to help ease their struggle. Sharing stories allowed me to connect with my community and lifted the sense of isolation that had taken over my life.

I realized that if I hoped to make a significant contribution to those around me, I needed to first restore my connection to my true self and my community in order to re-inject life into practicing the principles of healthy living.

Once I had regained both my life's desire and, more specifically, the desire to practice the principles of healthy living, I knew I needed to protect those precious gifts. These desires were vulnerable at first. I learned to protect them by carefully choosing my circle of influence and restoring my sense of faith in the wisdom of the universe.

As I reflect back on my moment to moment ability to handle the challenges, the few moments of peace I was able to muster, if only temporarily, were when I put faith in the wisdom of the universe. When I felt a sense of peace, I trusted that my challenges served purpose, that they were perfectly orchestrated to prepare me to ultimately fulfill my life's desire.

I trusted that the universe is both wise and efficient. I trusted that my father's death was all part of a bigger plan, which needed to happen just the way it did in order for those around him to experience the life we were meant to.

I choose to believe that if I had not sustained injuries in the car accident, I would never have explored physiotherapy or naturopathic medicine as a profession. I choose to believe that I was given the opportunity to gain a newfound strength by climbing out of the depths of despair to share that process with you.

I choose to believe that my life's desire is being fulfilled right under my nose—I just didn't always see it.

I am offering you an opportunity to take a gentler route. Explore your life's desires before tragedy strikes. If I am arriving too late, I may perhaps help you find peace after tragedy. One of the gifts you'll receive is the restoration of your life's desire and in turn a desire to practice the principles of healthy living.

> **To gain access to Endless Desire:**
>
> - Recognize the integral role that your health plays in fulfilling your life's desires.
>
> - Get in touch with your life's desire by connecting with your true self.
>
> - Express your life's desires through your connection to community.
>
> - Protect your life's desires by choosing your circle of influence wisely and maintaining your faith.

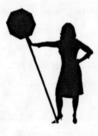

Destination III

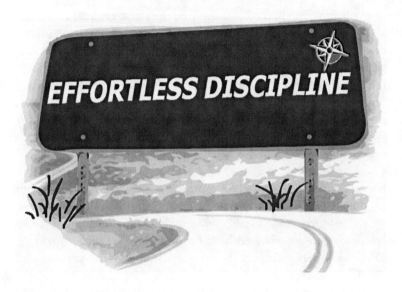

He who cannot change the very fabric of his thought will never be able to change reality.

—Anwar Sadat

When I ask my clients what stops them from looking and feeling their best, the third of the four most common stop signs I hear is, "I just don't seem to have the discipline." Discipline is the ability to consistently carry out the plans we create. This ability is absolutely essential when we want to turn our desires into reality. For the remainder of this book, when I use the term discipline I will be referring to discipline as it applies to self or self-discipline. What I've noticed in conversations with clients is that discipline has always been presented to them as something they learn to apply, not something they can develop.

But no one ever taught them how to develop the discipline they so desperately need. No one ever told them discipline could be effortless. When I reveal this idea to my clients, they breathe a sigh of relief, pull their chairs a little closer, and listen.

When our mind processes thoughts in an effective fashion, with the only acceptable outcome being our highest good, discipline arrives naturally and effortlessly. What I have found most effective in developing an effortless sense of discipline is to first build a strong foundation of self-value. Upon this foundation of self-value, we apply an effective method of creating strategies that enhance our lives. When we value ourselves, we are inclined to create life-enhancing strategies to meet our desires and are inspired to take action to fulfill our desires. When we are inspired to take action, we exercise an effortless sense of discipline.

Creating an effective strategy means that when we reflect, reason, analyze, and make decisions, we only accept outcomes that enhance our lives. When we make life-enhancing choices with respect to our health and follow through on them, we find ourselves practicing the principles of healthy living. Making constructive nutritional, activity-related, and other lifestyle choices are exactly what the principles of healthy living are all about.

Since we have the power to determine our thoughts, we ultimately have the power to choose one thought over another and dramatically impact our lives. When we value ourselves, we take pride in both our health and appearance. When we take pride in our health and appearance, we are inspired to invest in it. When we superimpose on that strong foundation of self-value an effective method for creating life-enhancing strategies, we find ourselves effortlessly turning our desires into reality. And when our actions are effortless, they are also free from stress.

As you live by the principles and use the concepts presented in this chapter, you will notice discipline appearing naturally in your life. You will find time where you thought there was none. You will set realistic, health-focused goals and take action to achieve them. You will feel the stress of your previous struggles just melt away.

This process ignites your desire to look and feel your best and creates effective strategies that transform your appearance by integrating the principles of healthy living into your life. Discipline need not be something you struggle to apply to your life; it is the natural product of a process you can learn and then relish. To begin the process we will make three quick rest stops where I introduce you to the principles that build self-value.

The Rest Stops

In *Seven Habits of Highly Effective People,* Stephen Covey reviewed two hundred years of success literature to find commonalities among the most successful individuals in history. He found that they used a principle-centered, character-based, inside-out approach to personal effectiveness. This approach involves using universal principles to guide our thoughts and behavior. The principles, he states, "are deep fundamental truths that have universal application.... Principles are guidelines for human conduct that are proven to have enduring, and permanent value."[11] Covey reminds us that each decision we make comes with its own set of consequences. We experience life-enhancing consequences if we live in harmony with universal principles, and life-diminishing ones if we don't.

Three universal principles—honesty, kindness, and fairness—are deep fundamental truths that, when used consistently and effectively, enhance our lives. When our lives are enhanced by staying true to these principles we build self-value. I have found it most effective to consider whether each decision we make is in harmony with the three principles. Taking these three quick rest stops as you navigate through life will help you to make choices that build self-value. When we value ourselves, we are inspired to consistently invest in our health and appearance, which happens naturally, without effort.

Honesty

Honesty is characterized by truth. To be honest is to tell the truth to the best of one's ability, and not to lie. I ask you, is a lie really a lie if you don't get caught? I have asked that question of many people, and there seems to be a consensus that it is. This is because the consequences of our actions happen whether someone finds out or not. So why do we still tell lies, ranging from tiny white ones to huge deceitful ones? Despite our beliefs, when we lie, even if we don't get caught, we are fooling no one.

Over the years I have come to recognize that lying has life-diminishing consequences far beyond what I could have imagined. Assuming you have a conscience, when you lie you know it. With each lie, we value ourselves a little less. It not only damages our relationship with ourselves, but with others as well. When lying becomes habitual, its life-diminishing consequences become crystal clear.

When I was a teenager, I took the recommendation of my uncle and enrolled in a personal development course offered by Context Associated called The Pursuit of Excellence that encouraged us to live in congruence with the statement, honesty really is the best policy. When we arrived the first morning, there was a tiny sign at the front of the room that very few, if any, noticed. It read, "Tell the

Truth." Every morning as we took our seats, we looked to the front of the room and the words grew larger and larger. On the last day they were so large that it was virtually impossible not to notice the sign, "TELL THE TRUTH."

It was interesting for me to hear others discuss the sign as it grew. It was as if their conscience was speaking to them. Having been raised in an environment that promoted openness and honesty, I was surprised by the effect of the sign. It raised the consciousness of truth so high that everyone was aware of the truthful environment and thus found it easy to express their truths. As participants shared their thoughts and feelings regarding the sign with the group, the room was bursting with honesty. I am convinced that this experience began a process for many, a process of enhancing lives and building self-value by staying true to the principle of honesty. I felt honored to be in the room to witness the power of the truth in its purest form.

Kindness

Kindness is characterized by friendliness, generosity, and consideration. When I think of kindness, two words come to mind: Uncle Norman. I refer to him as "the king of random acts of kindness." As I sift through the many memories I have, I cannot remember a time when he acted out of anything other than a pure desire to be kind and to give without expectation of receiving anything in return.

When I was still a child, chasing my Olympic dream, Uncle Norman joined the parents group of my gymnastics club on behalf of mine, who couldn't be there. He participated with the rigor of a parent, helping in any way he could. He even took some of his treasured stock-car racing trophies and replaced the little car on top with a gymnast and donated them to our club. When I visit his home, I am reminded that he is one of few that have been recognized for his incredible generosity in donations of blood to the Red Cross. When I leave I am hard pressed to make it out the door without a gift having been slipped into my pocket. These are only a small sample of the unending acts of kindness he delivers every day of his life.

His actions are focused on bringing a smile to the faces of those around him. I am sure he is not acutely aware of the tremendous impact his actions have on the lives of others. But when you give without expectation, as he does, you create an opportunity to build your self-value.

When I discuss the principle of kindness with my clients, most tell me that they believe kindness to be an integral part of our relationships with others, but few seem to be aware that kindness needs to be extended to their relationship with themselves. I hear stories of their generosity in support of others striving to improve their health, how they lend an ear, lend some money, and extend a hand to their family, friends, and lovers. It is less often that I hear stories of their self-kindness, especially in the realm of putting the time aside to focus on improving their own health and practicing the principles of healthy living. As a result their self-value, appearance, and health all suffer.

When I ask clients to treat themselves with kindness, I suggest things like preparing and consuming a healthy meal, going to the gym, taking a nap, setting aside time for self-reflection and self-awareness, taking time to read a book, take a bath, watch a movie, get a massage, or scheduling time for their favorite hobby.

I invite you to spend some time thinking of ways you can treat yourself with kindness and start implementing them right away.

Fairness

Fairness, or the ability to make judgments free from discrimination, is the third of three principles that build self-value. Being raised in a Christian household, fairness for me was best described by the Golden Rule, "Do unto others as you would have them do unto you" (Matthew 7:12). For many years, I thought that fairness was simply displayed through equality. Treating everyone equally required being nonjudgmental with respect to race, gender, age, appearance, abilities, and wealth, and exercising this equality would be deemed fair.

Because only we have direct access to our own thoughts, we have the privilege of knowing how we like to be treated. What I have noticed is that we are most inclined to treat others as we would like to be treated. I propose that true fairness is more than that. It involves consideration. Consideration requires that we listen empathetically, without judgment, in conversations with ourselves and with others. We collect all relevant information, as thoroughly and truthfully as possible, to hear the wants or needs of ourselves or another. Once we have a good idea, from another perspective, we can tailor our behavior to each situation we encounter. I propose that equality plus consideration equals fairness.

I would like to caution you to steer clear of a common pitfall I noticed while working with my clients. When faced with the life-diminishing behaviors of others, my clients offer understanding, patience, and forgiveness. Often, when faced with their own personal life-diminishing realizations regarding their own behavior, they hold themselves to unattainable standards. When they fail to meet these standards, they judge themselves as inadequate. When this self-judgment and resultant self-dissatisfaction is repeated it diminishes self-value. Remember, self-value is the foundation upon which to create strategies that enhance our lives, thereby opening the door to an effortless sense of discipline.

When I prescribe self-fairness to my clients, many of them ask me what I mean. It means saying no to life-diminishing choices that compromise their ability to practice the principles of healthy living, things that they would have otherwise said yes to. It means not holding themselves to unattainable standards and then judging themselves as inadequate. It is the belief in themselves that they deserve to be treated with honesty and kindness, regardless of gender, age, race, wealth, or appearance.

Don Miguel Ruiz, in his book *The Four Agreements,* tells us that the agreements we make with ourselves are the most important ones. Making and sticking to the agreements we make with ourselves regarding honesty, kindness, and fairness builds self-value. I invite you to strive to make, and keep, an agreement to use the principles of honesty, kindness, and fairness when creating strategies for yourself. With a foundation of self-value firmly in place, we next look to the concepts that I have found to be effective in shaping the creation of life-enhancing strategies. Consistently implementing this process provides access to an effortless sense of discipline.

The Car Wash

Millions of people are taking the initiative to improve and succeed in all aspects of life, including health, wealth, and relationships, in hopes of ultimately increasing the joy and happiness they experience. Getting to know ourselves better and acknowledging our vulnerabilities with the intent of enhancing our lives is the first step towards achieving those hopes. Improving our self-awareness is not, as some of my clients believe, a sign of weakness. In fact, it is exactly the opposite; it is a sign of strength. It takes strength and courage to honestly explore any aspect of our being and use this awareness to improve our lives.

There are three "cleansing" concepts that I have found to be most effective in creating strategies that are constructive to our lives: self-awareness, empowerment, and expectation. I will teach you an effective method of processing thoughts that will ensure that you create clean strategies, by which I mean only strategies that enhance your life. This clean and effective method begins by focusing on improving self-awareness. Once we have a better understanding of ourselves, we can use the concepts of empowerment and expectation to create strategies that enhance our lives.

What is necessary to change a person is to change his awareness of himself.
—Abraham Maslow

Self-Awareness

In *Seven Habits of Highly Effective People,* Covey defines self-awareness as "the ability to think about our every thought process," which "enables us to stand apart and examine even the way we 'see' ourselves." [11] Improving self-awareness is essential to the creation of lasting and multidimensional success. If used effectively, self-awareness provides access to personal growth, change, and evolution and ultimately enhances our lives.

When I question my clients regarding their self-awareness, they typically respond in one of two ways. Some are unaware that people even think about their thought process. I ask these individuals to consider that we have the freedom to use our thoughts to create both life-enhancing and life-diminishing strategies. Creating the former increases the likelihood that we meet our needs, wants, and desires in the future.

Other clients tell me that they do think about their thought process, but they choose not to venture into the realm of self-awareness because they are afraid to find out that what they are doing is wrong. Their biggest worry, they tell me, is that they would then need to change it. I encourage these individuals to see the process of improving self-awareness as an opportunity to get to know yourself better. Deepening awareness is the natural course of all long-term relationships, so why, I ask them, would they limit their relationship with themselves.

So how does one improve self-awareness? With education and unrelenting self-reflection is the answer. In his book *Think and Grow Rich,* Napoleon Hill provides an eloquent illustration of self-reflection. According to Hill, self-reflection can expose vulnerabilities that most individuals do not like to acknowledge, but this is essential if we want more from life than mediocrity.

He asks us to imagine that we ourselves are on trial and that we strive to play the role of all of those involved in the courtroom of our life. If we attempt to see things as the court and the jury, the prosecutor and the defense, the plaintiff and the defendant see them, we'll gain multiple perspectives.

Hill tells us to face facts truthfully and to question and reply to ourselves. When the trial is complete, we will know ourselves much better. If we cannot be an impartial judge during the trial, he encourages us to find someone else that knows us well to act as judge while we cross-examine ourselves.

Cultivating self-awareness does not need to be difficult. Often our circumstances show us where we need to begin. I learned a tip in my first Context Associated seminar that illustrates when to begin self-reflection. If you find yourself pointing your finger at someone, highlighting a behavior that irritates you, look down at your hand. When you point, your index finger may be pointing at the other party, but there are three fingers pointing back at you. I ask you to consider that your needs, wants or desires are not being fulfilled and that you would best be served by looking inward.

I challenge you, when you catch yourself pointing your finger, to begin reflecting on the issue that irritated you. How did you feel? Is this feeling easily triggered? Do the same feelings repeatedly arise? Remember, if you want to see changes on the outside, you first need to look inside. The next chapter is dedicated to processing our feelings so we can use them to create effective strategies in our lives.

People are disturbed not by things but by the view they take of them.

—*Epictetus*

Empowerment

In addition to improving self-awareness, what I have found to be most effective in creating life-enhancing strategies is to strive to place ourselves in a position of empowerment. I describe empowerment as a feeling of power within, the kind of feeling that encourages us to take the initiative to create strategies that improve the quality of our lives. The perspective we take, or how we choose to receive our circumstances, has a significant impact on our feeling of empowerment.

From the thoughts we think to the feelings we feel, from the actions we take to the spirit we radiate, every choice we make serves to either empower or disempower us. If the consequences of our choices serve to disempower us, they feed into a victim mentality and feelings of helplessness. This life-diminishing strategy both creates stress and prevents us from accessing an effortless sense of discipline.

During self-reflection it is helpful to recognize where we place ourselves in the empowerment spectrum. If we recognize that the choices we make serve to disempower us, its time to rework the strategy, refining our thoughts until we place ourselves in a position of empowerment.

There are five influential perspectives that I have found to be most effective in refining our thoughts. They all substantially increase the likelihood that we will place ourselves in a position of empowerment. Although these concepts are common in the realm of self-development I was first introduced to them when I participated in courses offered by Context Associated and Landmark Education Corporation. Keep in mind that the five perspectives are intertwined. Working together, they can help you create and maintain a position of empowerment.

Act vs. React

When we act, the thoughts we think, the feelings we feel, and the actions we take are derived from inside us. When we react, we are thinking, feeling, and taking action based on a response to something coming from the outside. When we react, we do not consciously choose our actions, we allow someone or something else to determine them. When we give our power away like this, we have placed ourselves in a position of disempowerment. If we are mindful of this choice in the moment, we can use it to modify our behavior on the spot. However, the awareness often comes during self-reflection after the event has passed and we can use it to make empowering choices in our future. It is important to steer clear of responding with a knee-jerk reaction triggered by emotion. When we react in the moment, this unprocessed response can be a source of regret. Ultimately, it allows others to determine our life instead of us.

I advocate acting as a chairperson in the meeting of our lives. We enter with our agenda prepared, knowing that what others say or how they behave will not be the sole determinant of our actions. It is most effective to direct our attention inward and sculpt our own lives. We protect our position of empowerment when we choose to act instead of simply reacting to our circumstances.

"Choose to" vs. "Have to"

How does it feel to you when you think you "have to" carry out a particular task? Now imagine that you "choose to" carry out that same task. Just the mere mention of having a choice completely changes the feeling. When we think that we have to, rather than choose to perform a particular task, it not only calls forth resistance but we deny ourselves personal accountability for our thoughts, feelings, and actions. Thinking that we have to, ultimately, takes away our power to choose. Making a choice takes back that same power. Remember, in every moment there is always a choice, and each choice is followed by its own unique set of consequences that are either life-enhancing or life-diminishing. Therefore, when you think thoughts and speak words, I encourage you to replace "I have to" and "I should" with words such as "I choose to", "I like to", "I want to" or "I am."

One Hundred Percent Accountable

I remember being taught that the sign of a good relationship is that it is fifty-fifty. To most, this seems both reasonable and fair. Then I became aware of the idea that it was in fact empowering to be 100 percent accountable in our relationships. When I began to explore the consequences of the fifty-fifty rule, I realized that it was in fact disempowering. First, it requires that we rely on someone else to achieve our goals, and second, when we meet those goals, we give away 50 percent of the credit. On the other hand, we would only shoulder 50 percent of the blame if we did not achieve our goals. On the surface, this appeared to be a fair trade, but as I processed these thoughts a little deeper, I realized that it takes away our power, 50 percent, to be exact. If we choose to be 100 percent accountable for our thoughts, feelings, actions, and ultimately our results, no matter what the circumstances, we take our lives into our own hands and have the power to shape them as we wish. This stops us from attempting to allocate fault or blame and thus is also empowering to our lives.

No Fault, No Blame

The perspective of "no fault, no blame" stops us from using fault and blame as reasons to avoid 100 percent accountability. In order to be fully empowered, we cannot blame others or ourselves for our circumstances. It is extremely helpful to listen without judgment and thereby gain a deeper level of compassion for the other person or a conflicting message in our internal dialogue. Once we see things as the other side does, we are less inclined to place blame. Then and only then can we begin to replace blame with empathy, understanding, forgiveness, and compassion.

I caution you to avoid the common pitfall of switching from blaming others to self-blame. Many of my clients state, "If it's not their fault, then it must be mine. It just has to be someone's fault." If we use the idea of "no fault, no blame" to see that things are just the way they are, nothing more and nothing less, we empower ourselves to move forward. I invite you to reflect on your past with the intention of building self-awareness and maintaining accountability but do not place blame.

Life Is Empty and Meaningless

At first, I found it hard to understand this idea. Is it not our purpose, I asked, to find meaning in life, meaning in joy, and meaning in suffering? In order to use this perspective effectively, I needed to reinterpret the meaning of the statement. Its purpose is to help me find an empowering perspective, which can only arise when we defuse our intense emotions. Reducing the intensity of our emotional responses brings things down to a manageable level where we choose to act rather than react, listen to others and ourselves without judgment, and focus on clearly identifying our feelings.

Simply put, the idea is a reminder not to take things personally. The second of four agreements discussed by Don Miguel Ruiz in his best-selling book, *The Four Agreements*, is just that: don't take anything personally. Sometimes we are so caught up in the intensity of our emotions we can't even see straight.

Our lives have only the meaning that we decide to place on them. There is no innate or inherent meaning in our experiences. It is our choice and our luxury to interpret and perceive things as we wish. I invite you to choose an interpretation that places you in a position of empowerment.

Expectation

The third concept that aids in creating strategies that enhance our lives is expectation. Many of my clients seem to have the expectation that life, and particularly their health, should be easier than it is, or at least it should not be so difficult. The word *expect* implies which means that we have judged the matter at hand. I don't pretend to know where this expectation comes from, but I do understand the repercussions of its use. The more we expect, the more intense are the feelings we experience when those expectations are unfulfilled.

It has been my experience that when we have a preconceived expectation of a particular outcome, we are more inclined to blame others in order to evade accountability for our actions. Many of my clients spend valuable time venting and complaining that they have been cheated in some way when they didn't get the outcome they expected. When they designate time here, they are investing significant amounts of energy resisting what is.

Letting go of expectation is a simple way to diminish the feelings that arise when our expectations are unfulfilled. It frees up time and energy that would have otherwise been invested in defusing the intense feelings when our expectations were not met. I am not suggesting that we sweep our feelings under the carpet. In fact, I have dedicated the majority of the next chapter to emotional awareness and effective emotional management. I am suggesting we dedicate an appropriate amount of time to this process, because once we have identified our feelings, we can turn our attention to forgiveness and compassion. And then we can ponder the important questions: Where can I go from here? How can I be proactive? Why have these circumstances entered my life? What is my lesson?

Think Your Way There

With his popular motivational technique, neuroassociative conditioning, Tony Robbins is recognized for making Neuro-Linguistic Programming (NLP) famous. NLP explores how our language influences our mind, how our language affects our perception, and in turn how our perception influences our behavior. In the early 1990s, I participated in an introductory NLP course and found it not only interesting but also extremely powerful.

Since we choose the thoughts we think and the words we speak, we have the power to create strategies that enhance our lives. This is how we participate in the creation of our reality. So if we want to make change in our lives, we begin by using language that matches our desires. As a result, we can change our circumstances when we start changing our thoughts. When we create life-enhancing strategies and then take action to make those strategies a reality, we improve the likelihood of successful manifestation.

We all know individuals who have changed their relationships, jobs, homes, marital status, material items, hair, and even appearance in hopes of bringing change into their lives. Then they realize their lives haven't changed in the way that they had hoped, because what they had hoped to leave behind follows them. The only way to make real change in our lives is to start changing the way we think.

In summary, creating a healthy sense of self-value and life-enhancing strategies leaves us with a gift. This gift is an effortless sense of discipline, because it compels us to take action towards our highest good.

My Road to Effortless Discipline

Once I had taken down my first two stop signs, the lack of energy and the lack of desire to nurture my health, I shifted my focus towards restoring discipline. In initially dealing with my challenges, I had lost the discipline to practice the principles of healthy living. With my sights set on reintegrating the principles of healthy living into my life, I began to participate consistently in my own personal development, striving to improve my self-awareness through education and self-reflection. I read books, enrolled in seminars, and engaged in discussions to acquire and then put into practice what I learned.

I began exploring the principles that my family had instilled in me when I was a child. Honesty, kindness, and fairness made their way to the forefront of my mind as I began to apply them to my life. I realized that my self-value had been to some degree tied to my accomplishments and to my relationship with family. After my sense of stability had been shattered, I knew I needed to rebuild it from the ground up, filling all the cracks in the foundation through adherence to the principles of honesty, kindness, and fairness. I needed to ensure that I was being honest with both myself and others regarding my thoughts, feelings, and physical state of health. I struggled with the feelings of disappointment surrounding my inability to achieve my career goals and my athletic and personal aspirations. I struggled to respond honestly when asked to share my feelings of sadness and disappointment with others. It was like rubbing salt in a wound every time I spoke of them. At the time, I didn't feel inspired to share my struggles with anyone.

Attempting to put my shortcomings into words was painful; it was like I had lost in the battle against life's circumstance.

As I reflected on myself with kindness in mind, I was reminded to be considerate and patient with myself and allow myself time to process my thoughts and feelings, time to grieve and heal. As I reflected on myself with fairness in mind, I was reminded to avoid self-judgment for what I viewed as shortcomings. It was unfair to hold myself to a standard that I could not at that point attain. I reminded myself that self-value is not tied solely to achieving my goals. Goals are milestones we set to direct our life, something we move towards. I reminded myself that I couldn't plan my personal route in life in its entirety. And I reminded myself to trust in the wisdom of the universe and maintain enough flexibility to be prepared for the landslides and floods that life presents.

When I struggled the most, I tended to create life-diminishing strategies. I thought that since my career aspirations were destroyed, I would not enjoy my work, make enough money, or attain the freedom I desired. Since my personal aspirations were crushed, I would not get married and have children, because I could not bear the thought of doing so without my father. He would not be there to walk me down the aisle or be a grandfather to my children.

Losing someone I loved was an experience that changed my life in an instant, with a nauseating sense of permanence. It drastically altered my perspective, changed my priorities, and forced me to assess my life from a completely different place. But, I knew that I had the freedom of choosing to create life-enhancing or life-diminishing strategies based on that perspective.

I spent time in self-reflection, listening to my stories without judgment, hoping to gain a better understanding of who I was, particularly when faced with adversity. Would I hold true to my beliefs and use the concepts such as empowerment and expectation? It was a clear picture of my life's desire that gave me the strength to focus on creating strategies that enhanced my life.

After my initial reaction to circumstance, I focused on making empowering choices. I began consciously acting instead of reacting. I replaced the words, "I have to" with "I choose to." Even though I was only a passenger in my car accident, I chose to be 100 percent accountable for my circumstances, thus allowing me to no longer blame the drivers and instead focus on healing. I believed that the drivers did the best they could under the circumstances at the time.

I noticed that the more tightly I held onto expectations, the more strongly I felt my disappointment. Initially, I held the expectation that I should not have had to suffer injury or the loss of my career, athletic ability, and personal aspirations. I held the expectation that my father should not have died so young, that he should have walked me down the aisle and been a grandfather to my children. Letting go of these expectations and stopping "shoulding" myself was freeing for me. My feelings of disappointment began to lift. I spent time pondering where I could go from here, how I could be proactive, and why these circumstances had entered my life. One of my most difficult achievements in the realm of empowerment was to use the perspective that life is empty and meaningless. I needed to reframe my perspective in order to see the value in it. I made an effort not to take things personally. I learned to see my life with much more clarity. Once applied, this perspective defused the intensity of my emotions, allowing me to act and not react.

As I began using the principles and concepts described above to create strategies that enhanced my life, I noticed my life's circumstance change right in front of my eyes. By changing my thought process, my life began to move in the direction of my desires.

To gain access to Effortless Discipline:

- Build a strong sense of self-value by living by the following principles:
    o   Be honest with yourself and others.
    o   Be kind to yourself and others.
    o   Be fair to yourself and others.
- Use these concepts to create strategies that enhance your life:
    o   Continually strive to improve your self-awareness.
    o   Let go of expectation.
    o   Place yourself in a position of empowerment.
    o   Remember that you manifest what you think.

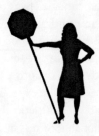

Destination IV

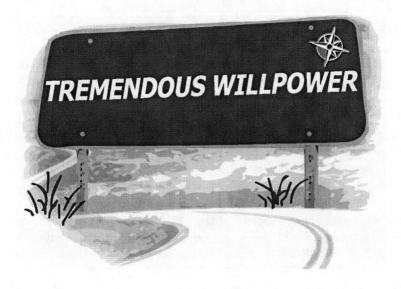

Strength does not come from physical capacity it comes from an indomitable will.

—Mahatma Gandhi

When I ask my clients what stops them from looking and feeling their best, the last of the four most common stop signs I hear is, "I just don't seem to have the willpower." My clients share stories of how they struggle to say no to things that they know sabotage their dreams. They tell me of pulling into the drive-through of a fast-food restaurant when they had intended to go home and prepare a nutritious meal. They tell of intending to have one helping of food at dinner but instead taking three. They tell of intending to go to the gym but deciding to watch a movie instead of exercising. They tell me how one glass of wine with dinner somehow turns into a whole bottle. Finally, they share how they planned to go to bed at ten but found themselves watching infomercials until two in the morning.

So how do we access the tremendous willpower needed to avoid sabotaging our intentions? To simplify the answer, if we break the word willpower into two parts, will and power, we note that will is the mental faculty by which we deliberately choose a course of action and power is the ability to act effectively. So when I use the word willpower, I refer to the ability to effectively and deliberately choose a course of action. To achieve our intended results, then, the power of our will needs to be exercised without obstruction. We all have access to tremendous willpower; we just, at times, choose to obstruct it.

There are areas in your life where the power of your will acts without even noticing. When you decide on a course of action that fulfills your daily needs and long-term goals with ease and grace you are accessing your power of will. But there may be areas in your life where this is difficult. For example, you may find it easy to make healthy nutritional choices but struggle to stay active. You may find it easy to stay active but struggle to make healthy food choices. You may find it easy to say no to alcohol but hard to say no to cake.

So what makes willpower easily accessible in one case and difficult in another? When we struggle to access our willpower, it is because we are experiencing conflicting messages in our internal dialogue. For example, when we are offered a piece of cake, one voice inside us says "yes please" and the other says "no thank you." When faced with situations such as this we attempt to use our willpower to reconcile the conflict, failing to realize that the very predicament we are in actually obstructs it. Herein lies the struggle.

The intensity of struggle we feel is based on how far apart the conflicting messages really are. The farther apart, the greater the internal struggle. To defuse this struggle, we resolve the conflict. For example, if we plan to exercise at noon three days per week and if, when noon arrives, we have no new conflicting message, we carry out that plan with ease. On the other hand, if we consider a new and conflicting message to forfeit the exercise when noon arrives, we feel the struggle between fulfilling our plan and sabotaging it.

When we feel this struggle, it is an indication that we need to resolve the conflict by using effective mental and emotional management. The most effective way I have found is to prevent it from occurring in the first place. Whether we are looking for prevention or moment-to-moment management, we look to our emotions for direction. The ability to identify and manage our emotions is critical if we want to resolve our struggles efficiently and effectively. Yet the idea of emotional awareness and effective emotional management seems to be unfamiliar in today's world.

In practice, when I nudge my way into the emotional realm of my clients' health, I often meet a subtle resistance, discomfort, or uneasiness. When I ask them to describe their feelings and how they manage them in their everyday lives, I am met with a blank stare. Breaking the stare, they might ask, "What do you mean?" Or they might say, "I don't know" or "No one has ever asked me that before." So how did we get to a place where the idea of emotional management is lost in the abyss?

Our Emotional Climate

Up until the mid-1990s, there was little value placed on emotions in general, but especially in the workplace. Consequently, few of us have been exposed to effective methods of identifying and managing our emotions. By publishing his book *Emotional Intelligence* in 1995, Daniel Goleman, PhD, popularized the term "emotional intelligence," which he defined as the ability to know and manage your feelings effectively. Goleman revealed that our EQ (emotional quotient) is a stronger predictor of success than our IQ, even in the workplace.

Shortly thereafter, Candace Pert, PhD, published *Molecules of Emotion,* in which she shares her discovery of scientific links between the mind and the body. Based upon years of research, she demonstrates that our emotions trigger the release of molecules that flow throughout the body, directly affecting our state of health and disease. She shows how stress disturbs the body's natural healing response by preventing molecules from flowing where they are needed for processes such as breathing, blood flow, immunity, digestion, and elimination.

What we learn from Goleman and Pert is that effective emotional management has a direct positive impact on not only successfully achieving our goals, but also easing our struggles to improve our overall state of health.

If you have happy thoughts, then you make happy molecules.

—Deepak Chopra

Reflecting on Your Trip

Marshall Rosenberg, PhD, in his book *Nonviolent Communication,* eloquently describes human beings as always acting in an attempt to meet their needs and values. He advocates that we become consciously aware of what we are perceiving, feeling, and wanting so that we have a better chance of creating strategies that will meet our needs and values in the future. Rosenberg's process for creating nonviolent communication is very similar to the process I use to resolve conflicting internal dialogue.

The key to resolving conflicting internal dialogue lies in our ability to identify and effectively manage our emotions. When we act in a manner that does not meet our needs, our emotions signal our discontent. Feelings are our hearts' way of letting us know we have reacted to an experience. Not unlike the signs and symptoms from our body, feelings are messages from our hearts that are calling out for our help. Our feelings not only let us know when our needs are not being met, they are also the force that drives us to meet our needs. What I have found to be most effective when it comes to emotional awareness—the component of self-awareness that specifically focuses on our feelings—is focusing on self-reflection. During self-reflection we strive to notice whether what we say and do is enhancing our lives or not, without judgment. In all my years of study, no matter what the source, there has been a constant theme regarding judgment. It is damaging to our relationships and our self-value. When we self-reflect without judgment, noticing whether our lives have been enhanced or not, we can acknowledge and then identify feelings that come up. These feelings are a response to our unfulfilled needs.

Many of my clients struggle to identify their feelings, and when they do, they are often uncomfortable feeling the full spectrum of their emotions. Part of the difficulty in identifying our emotions lies in our lack of familiarity with words that identify specific feelings. Rosenberg provides a list of emotions that we are likely to feel when our needs are being met and a list of ones we are likely to feel when they are not. I encourage you to use these words to improve your emotional vocabulary so that you may be more specific when identifying your emotions in the future. Many of my clients are preoccupied with emotional hygiene, focused only on acknowledging "positive" emotions and ignoring the "negative" ones in an attempt to use the power of positive thinking to their advantage. I invite you to regard feelings as neither good nor bad. They just *are* and each arises with a message and an opportunity for us to enhance our lives.

Embracing the Opportunity

Holding on to anger is like holding on to a hot coal with the intent of throwing it at someone else; you are the one who gets burned.

—*Buddha*

When during self-reflection we notice that the choice we made did not enhance our life and have identified the emotions that arose when our needs were not met, we have an opportunity to forgive ourselves. When we recognize that our efforts were simply an attempt to enhance our life, even if it was not successful, we forgive.

When we forgive, we replace our feelings of disappointment over our choices with compassion. I like to use the saying "we did the best we could under the circumstances at the time" to free ourselves from physical, mental and emotional suffering. When we recognize that we were only acting in an attempt to fulfill a need, we forgive ourselves without effort. It is in forgiveness that we find release from the pain of past choices.

Releasing pain is the most powerful opportunity we have for healing. Forgiving and freeing ourselves from pain allows us to create new and different strategies that have a better chance of meeting our needs in the future and in turn enhancing our lives. Some of our strongest emotions are generated from feelings of hurt and lack of forgiveness. To sever the hold that lack of forgiveness has on us, we lift its fingers, one by one, until the strength of the grip is broken. When we complete this process, we experience peace of mind, which lets us know that we have forgiven ourselves.

Emotions that arise when our needs are not met by the choices we make serve a very important purpose. They act as a signal that we have reacted to something and show us exactly where to start to identify the underlying need that has not been met. Identifying the underlying need provides us with a foundation upon which to create a new strategy to meet our need. When our new strategy is created directly from our insight into the need, it's easy to design one that meets that need in the future.

When we create a new and different strategy using the process described above, it has a better chance of fulfilling our needs. By repeating this process over and over again we learn to meet our needs by creating strategies that enhance our lives. What I have found to be effective is to use the principles and concepts I described in the chapter on effortless discipline to create a new effective strategy to meet our needs and enhance our lives. Running the potential strategy through this process creates a life-enhancing strategy. Each time we repeat this process it minimizes the chance that we will experience conflicting messages of internal dialogue in the future. When we minimize the appearance of conflicting messages in our life, temptation has no choice but to give its power back to us. When you feel this tremendous power of will, it's easy to make choices that enhance your life, such as practicing the principles of healthy living.

When, you might ask, will you find the time to put this process into action? Noticing the impact of our choices, identifying feelings and their underlying needs, and creating new strategies can be done under all sorts of circumstances: during the creation of art, music, and literature, through conversing, or just by reflecting on ourselves in our own minds.

Personally, I find it is in the maintenance tasks like exercising, driving, showering, cooking, cleaning, and doing laundry that I find time in my busy schedule to self-reflect. When I ask my clients when they find it most convenient to self-reflect, many tell me they just don't have the time. Some say it's due to demanding work or family schedules. Others spend their time watching TV, playing computer games, surfing the Internet, or reading magazines or newspapers. In other words, they occupy their minds with anything other than self-reflection.

Overfilling the Gas Tank

We all know that if we don't clean the home, it gets dirty. If we don't do the laundry, it piles up. We know that maintenance is required in all aspects of life if we hope to achieve some level of success. Our feelings are no different. The danger in failing to identify our emotions and their underlying needs is that we are less equipped to forgive and then create a new and different strategy that has a better chance of meeting our need in the future.

This buildup of emotions from unfulfilled needs and lack of forgiveness initiates the stress cascade, depleting our overall state of health and increasing our risk of acquiring chronic disease. Acknowledging our emotions and using them to meet our needs in the future enhances our lives by improving our health and our happiness. If we have not yet accessed these skills, we suffer. In his book *The Seat of the Soul,* Gary Zukav reminds us that when we suffer, we look elsewhere for fulfillment.

As we attempt to fulfill our emotional needs, it is a common strategy to turn to the overconsumption of food. But food is not capable of meeting emotional needs. This strategy, at best, provides a temporary feel-good solution but has devastating long-term effects on our self-value, our health, and ultimately our appearance.

To break this cycle of overconsumption, he suggests we stop overconsuming long enough to notice the feelings that surface when we abstain. This provides a window of opportunity to identify the underlying need, forgive ourselves, and create a new strategy to meet our emotional needs. When our lives are enhanced because our needs are fulfilled, the drive to overconsume just melts away, allowing our tremendous power of will to shine through.

Learning to Coast

In his book *Blink: The Power of Thinking without Thinking,* Malcolm Gladwell, PhD, compares our unconscious brain to a computer-processing chip. Pure conscious thinking, he says, is actually limiting. It does not allow us to tap into the wonder of our unconscious brain. Trying to function without utilizing this part of our brain is like trying to solve a complicated mathematical equation without using a calculator or like not using a search engine when looking for a Web page on the Internet.

Our unconscious brain functions involuntarily, whether we make an effort to influence it or not. It works day and night and never gets tired. It does not need time to recharge. I have found it effective to input wants and needs and then sleep on it. Let it simmer, stew, and brew like a Crock-Pot. Our job is to put in the raw ingredients and then leave it. When we come home from a hard day's work and lift the lid, there is a succulent meal, ready and waiting for us.

We are in charge of selecting the recipe and preparing the ingredients that make up the dish that we call our future. The ingredients are the thoughts and feelings we derive from identifying our wants and needs. To ensure that they are of the highest quality, I recommend using the self-reflective process described above, and then hand them over to the computer chip of our soul to enrich the process. When they return to our conscious brain for interpretation and integration, we notice that our desires begin to manifest themselves with much less work.

My Road to Tremendous Willpower

There are hundreds of examples I could share with you that demonstrate how to apply the information I have presented in this chapter regarding effective mental and emotional management. I chose the following example because I know, from my experience with clients, how common it is to struggle with potentially devastating long-term effects on our health. I hope that seeing this information in action helps ease your struggle as it did mine.

Following the extreme challenges in my life, I was faced with such intense emotions that they literally rocked the foundation of my being. I knew that I needed some guidance to work through them. The counselor I chose came highly recommended and I felt that I benefited from my sessions, but it wasn't until recently, when I read *Nonviolent Communication* by Marshall Rosenberg, that I identified my style of emotional management. I had somehow, through the course of my life, learned to use my feelings, most notably the feelings associated with the challenges in my life, as an indication to focus my attention there.

Following my car accident, on the advice of my team physician, I ceased all athletic activity, and for the first time in my life I struggled to maintain the healthy body composition that I had spent my whole life developing. Due to a long and intense history of participation in elite sports, I developed a fast metabolism, a large amount of muscle mass, and an equally large appetite. At first, I continued to consume the same number of calories as I had before my accident, but I now failed to burn them at the same rate.

This relative overconsumption of food was directly responsible for my slow and steady weight gain. I resisted the idea of reducing my caloric intake because I associated that with defeat. I wanted to act, not react, to my circumstances. I wanted to fulfill my career goals and personal aspirations. I wanted so desperately to hold on to my old life, the one where I was in charge, where I was happy, and where my desires seemed to be realized without effort.

Since I lacked the knowledge, experience, clarity, and focus I have today, my struggle, though diminishing slowly, continued. I created new life-enhancing strategies to improve my physical pain and energy levels so I could return to exercise. Each time I created a strategy, I attempted to improve upon the last, reworking it until finally a sense of peace permeated my heart. That is when I recognized my need for autonomy, the freedom to choose my plans for fulfilling my goals.

When I look back on my struggle, I see the conflicting messages in my internal dialogue. One message was to reduce my caloric intake until I was able to return to the activities that would allow me to burn them off. The second message was to continue my relative overconsumption of food attempting to avoid defeat. These conflicting messages prevented me from finding easy access to my power of will to make the life-enhancing choice of reducing my caloric intake. I noticed that my choice to listen to the second message certainly did not enhance my life. My behavior was in fact directly responsible for the undesirable shift in my body composition.

The feeling that surfaced when I reflected on my behavior was fear. I was afraid of losing my freedom of choice to continue exercising and eating as I once had. My underlying need that I was so desperately attempting to fulfill was autonomy. I wanted to choose what form of exercise I would participate in and how much time I would spend doing it. I wanted to choose what foods I would eat and how many calories I would consume.

Fortunately, forgiveness arrived when I recognized that maintaining my caloric consumption resulting in the subsequent shift in my body composition was simply an attempt to meet my need for autonomy and freedom of choice. This self-forgiveness appeared naturally without effort. The emotional pain that had infiltrated my being as a result of my car accident began to disappear as I recognized my tremendous effort to protect one of my most precious gifts, my freedom. One of the greatest gifts I gave to myself was the gift of compassion. I recognized that I did the best I could under the circumstances at the time.

With my newfound forgiveness, I was able to go back to the drawing board and create a new strategy to meet my need for autonomy. Fortunately, this time it would be a life-enhancing one. I replaced the words "I have to" with "I choose to" balance my caloric intake with my activity levels, thus filling both my need for autonomy and my need to nurture my body by maintaining a healthy body composition.

The Open Road

As I continued to live by the principles, concepts, perspectives, ideas, and philosophies presented in this book, my desires began to materialize right in front of my eyes. To my utter surprise, the dean of the school of dentistry finally offered me the opportunity to pursue a career as a dentist. Ironically, I declined his offer as my needs and aspirations had completely changed through my challenges and the resultant personal growth. Individuals began to appear in my life that provided the physical, mental, emotional, and spiritual expertise that I craved at my most vulnerable point.

I never returned to elite sporting activities. Instead I discovered new physical activities that gave me tremendous personal satisfaction. I now identified with my unique gifts and talents and created stronger relationships with friends, family, and the colleagues who supported me in my decision to use those gifts. The peak of my personal evolution arrived in the form of my role of helping others fulfill their life's desires. The ultimate gift I gave myself materialized as the opportunity to share my story with you. My dream now is to be an usher to those at personal crossroads, to help others celebrate their own unique gifts and open the road ahead for them.

To gain access to Tremendous Willpower:

- Remember that tremendous willpower is a natural state, operating without obstruction.

- Remember that the power of will is diminished when it is obstructed by conflicting internal dialogue.

- Acknowledge that feelings are not good and bad, they all have purpose.

- Spend time in self-reflection to notice what is not enhancing your life and identify feelings that arise when you do.

- Ensure that you forgive yourself for the choices you have made.

- Identify the underlying need that has not been fulfilled.

- If you find yourself excessively consuming food, stop, identify your feelings and the underlying need that is not being met, and focus on creating a new life-enhancing strategy to fulfill those needs.

- Remember how easy it can be to have your needs and desires manifest.

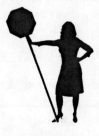

The Ultimate Destination—
The Healthier, Sexier You!

True nobility isn't about being better than someone else. It's about being better than you used to be.

—Wayne Dyer

Passion is the driving force behind all of our actions that are free from resistance. Trying to make our journey without passion is like planning a road trip to the peak of a mountain without having a motor under the hood. Passion is what compels us to fulfill our desires, desires of all kinds. A passion for health compels us to integrate the principles of healthy living into our lives. It is the natural result of minimizing stress by choosing the most efficient and effective route on a journey through all dimensions of our health.

Ladies and Gentlemen, Start Your Engines!

If you haven't done so already, it's time to look carefully at yourself to identify and remove what's stopping you from gaining access to any or all of the four essential destinations on your road to looking and feeling your best.

You are now in a position to begin taking down your stop signs and consciously create a new way of managing your health. You will no longer wonder why you struggled to look and feel your best. You will no longer be satisfied with operating on autopilot, as you may have in the past. And you will no longer struggle to overcome bad habits.

The time has come to optimize your physical health and restore an unlimited sense of energy. Focus on integrating the principles of healthy living into your life. If your body is calling out for help and your fatigue is not easily alleviated, you may require assessment from a qualified health care professional.

The time has come to optimize your spiritual health and restore an endless sense of desire. Focus on connecting with your life's desire and understanding the integral role that health plays in fulfilling this desire.

The time has come to optimize your mental health and restore an effortless sense of discipline. Strive to live by the principles that build self-value and use the concepts that create strategies that enhance your life.

The time has come to optimize your emotional health and restore your tremendous power of will. Strive to resolve conflicting messages in your internal dialogue so that they will no longer pull you in two separate directions, thus giving you a sense of peace.

I encourage you to direct your efforts towards designing your own personal road map, one that is devoid of detours and stop signs. Once you have visited all four essential destinations and tapped into your passion for health, nurturing it feels like a hobby. When your health feels like a hobby, it's easy to practice the principles of healthy living. When it's easy to practice the principles of healthy living, your physical appearance falls right into place.

When you live in integrity with these principles, you will arrive at your final destination: the healthier, sexier you. And this will let you know, loud and clear, that you are finally able to Stop Being Stopped.

Staying on Course

The way to gain a good reputation is to endeavor to be what you desire to appear.

—*Socrates*

Integrity is a firm adherence to a code of especially moral or artistic values. I am sure that you are well aware that for this journey to be effective, it is important to strive to live with integrity in accordance with what you have learned. When you encounter bumps on the road, as we all do, please do not quit. Take note of your vulnerabilities, self-reflect, learn from your experience, and use that knowledge to move forward with even greater momentum.

At the end of this chapter I have included a "Checklist for Staying on Course." I urge you to use it to maneuver around the bumps. Tear it out and place it where you have easy access to it, so that when struggles arise, you can use it to avoid lengthy detours and unnecessary stop signs.

Remember, no matter what route you choose, be patient, because learning how best to nurture your health to a sexier self is an exciting, lifelong journey! When you live in integrity, adhering to the philosophies described in each of the four essential destinations, you will have no trouble achieving your health dreams.

So, I ask that you go forth with integrity. Live with vigor, follow your vision, and take control of your destiny—let nothing stand in your way!

To gain access to Your Passion for Health:

- Be sure that you are free of fatigue and are practicing the principles of healthy living, so that you may access Unlimited Energy.
- Recognize the integral role that your health plays in nurturing your spirit, so that you may access Endless Desire.
- Strive to live by the principles that build self-value and concepts that create effective strategies that enhance your life, so that you may access Effortless Discipline.
- Resolve conflicting internal dialogue through effective emotional management, so that you may access Tremendous Willpower.
- Live your life with integrity.

A Checklist for Staying on Course

When you are struggling to find passion for health, identify the dimension of your health that you are struggling with and then refer to the "destination" below that is associated with that dimension and focus your efforts there.

When you are struggling to find an unlimited sense of energy:

- Take steps to diffuse your stress effectively by focusing your efforts on the dimension of your health where you believe the stress is rooted.
- Review the principles of healthy living and ask yourself, "Where can I improve with respect to living these principles?"
- Complete the Fatigue Test

- Review the medical conditions that apply to you, looking specifically for signs and symptoms that you experience.
- Take action to optimize your physical health by seeking appropriate treatment from a qualified health care professional for any signs, symptoms, or conditions that you suspect you have.

When you are struggling to find an endless sense of desire:

- Recognize the integral role that your health plays in fulfilling your life's desires.
- Get in touch with your life's desires by connecting with your true self.
- Express your life's desires through your connection to community.
- Protect your life's desires by choosing your circle of influence wisely and maintaining your faith.

When you are struggling to find an effortless sense of discipline:

- Build a strong sense of self-value by living by the following principles:
  - Be honest with yourself and others.
  - Be kind to yourself and others.
  - Be fair to yourself and others.
- Use these concepts to create strategies that enhance your life:
  - Continually strive to improve your self-awareness.
  - Let go of expectation.
  - Place yourself in a position of empowerment.
  - Remember that you manifest what you think.

When you are struggling to find a tremendous sense of willpower:

- Remember that tremendous willpower is a natural state, operating without obstruction.
- Remember that the power of will is diminished when it is obstructed by conflicting internal dialogue.
- Acknowledge that feelings are not good and bad, they all have purpose.
- Spend time in self-reflection to notice what is not enhancing your life and identify feelings that arise when you do.

- Ensure that you forgive yourself for the choices you have made.
- Identify the underlying need that has not been fulfilled.
- If you find yourself excessively consuming food, stop, identify your feelings and the underlying need that is not being met, and focus on creating a new life-enhancing strategy to fulfill those needs.
- Remember how easy it can be to have your needs and desires manifest.

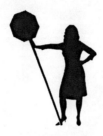

New Horizons

Whatever you can do, or dream you can do, begin it.
Boldness has genius, power, and magic in it.

—*attributed to Goethe*

I have no doubt that many of you, after getting a small taste of this material, have developed a hunger for more. Acquiring this type of knowledge, growth, and development can become seductive. As far as information on the topics discussed in this book goes, I have only exposed you to the tip of the iceberg; this type of information runs broad and deep. If you are interested in continuing your education, you can visit my Web site at http://stopbeingstopped.com. Depending on your style of learning and individual needs, you can choose how you would like to turn the information in my book into your reality.

Once you experience the power of personal development, you will be compelled to engage in this lifelong learning process, because how you feel when you invest in yourself is rich! My parting wish is that I have helped you gain access to the four destinations that tap into your passion for health and that, finally, you will have stopped being stopped!

Remember,

It's easy to walk on water once you know where the rocks are.

—*Anonymous*

Giving You the GREEN LIGHT!

Dr. Karen Lee Paquette
karen@stopbeingstopped.com

About the Author

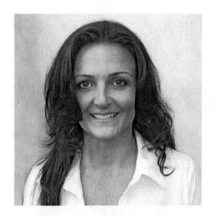

Dr. Karen Lee Paquette, BS, BSPT, RCAMT, ND, CCC is a respected Physical Therapist, Naturopathic Doctor, and Life Coach who has dedicated her life to learning, teaching, and practicing the principles of healthy living. For the past five years, she has been an Associate Professor, Curriculum Consultant, and Clinical Supervisor at the Canadian College of Naturopathic Medicine in Toronto.

Dr. Paquette holds both a BS in Zoology and a BS in Physical Therapy from the University of British Columbia, an RCAMT from the Canadian Academy of Manipulative Therapy, an ND, doctorate diploma, from The Canadian College of Naturopathic Medicine, and a CCC, Certified Comprehensive Coach, from Comprehensive Coaching U.

Dr. Paquette comes inimitably qualified, having acquired a set of unique personal and professional credentials that enable her to view your health, from a completely new and innovative perspective.

Since 1994, she has been teaching her clients the principles of healthy living, helping them change their lives one at a time through the development and operation of some of the most successful client programs in her field. In addition to her work locally, Dr. Paquette traveled extensively as a personal physical therapist of World Champion and four-time Olympian, David Ford.

Inspired to extend her impact globally, Karen—employing the moniker, The GO Doctor—has written *Stop Being Stopped: The GO Doctor's Guide to Unleashing the Healthier, Sexier You*! Currently she offers continuing education designed to pick up where her book leaves off, providing creative approaches and resources that help individuals turn the principles in her book into reality.

Your Medical Guide

The Fatigue Test

Note

The majority of the test questions are drawn from a *Health Appraisal Questionnaire* designed by Lyra Heller and Mike Katke listed in the selected bibliography.

Warning

This test is not a complete appraisal of your overall health. It is specifically designed to help you narrow down the systems of your body that are calling out for help. The results will determine which category(s) of fatigue or stress-related disorders to review.

Directions

This test asks how you have been feeling **during the last four months.** Take all the time you need to complete it.

For each item, circle the number that best describes your symptoms.

0 = No or Rarely. You have never experienced the symptom, or the symptom is familiar to you, but you perceive it as insignificant (monthly or less).

1 = Occasionally. The symptom comes, goes, and is linked in your mind to stress, diet, fatigue, or some identifiable trigger.

4 = Often. The symptom occurs two to three times per week or with a frequency that bothers you enough that you would like to do something about it.

8 = Frequently. The symptom occurs four or more times per week, or you are aware of the symptom every day, or it occurs with regularity on a monthly or cyclical basis.

Some questions require a yes or no response.

0 = No

8 = Yes

Other items require circling a number that describes how frequently you engage in a lifestyle behavior.

Please use the numerical system above.

Scoring

If you scored less than ten in all sections, congratulations! Please turn directly to "The Principles of Healthy Living" on page fourteen to maintain or optimize your good health right now.

If you scored over ten in any section, please consult the appropriate section of "The Many Faces of Fatigue" following the test and review the medical conditions to determine if any apply to you, paying particular attention to the signs and symptoms. Then, when finished, please turn directly to the "Scheduling a Tune-up" section on page eighteen to find out what you can do right away to continue improving your health.

Part I. Digestive Health	
Section A	
1. Indigestion; food repeats on you after you eat	(0) 1 4 8
2. Excessive burping, belching, or bloating following meals	0 (1) 4 8
3. Stomach spasms and cramping during or after eating	(0) 1 4 8
4. A sensation that food just sits in your stomach creating uncomfortable fullness, pressure and bloating during or after a meal	(0) 1 4 8
5. Bad taste in your mouth	(0) 1 4 8
6. Small amounts of food fill you up immediately	(0) 1 4 8
7. Skip meals or eat erratically because you have no appetite	(0) 1 4 8
8. When massaging under your rib cage on your left side, there is pain, tenderness, or soreness	(0) 1 4 8
9. Indigestion, fullness or tension in your abdomen is delayed, occurring 2-4 hours after eating a meal	(0) 1 4 8
10. Lower abdominal discomfort is relieved with the passage of gas or with a bowel movement	(0) 1 4 8
11. The consistency or form of your stool changes (e.g., from narrow to loose) within the course of the day	0 (1) 4 8
12. Stool odor is embarrassing	(0) 1 4 8
13. Undigested food in your stool	(0) 1 4 8
14. Diarrhea (frequent loose, watery stool)	0 (1) 4 8
15. Discomfort, pain, or cramps in your colon (lower abdominal area)	(0) 1 4 8
16. Emotional stress or eating raw fruits and vegetables causes abdominal bloating, pain, cramps, or gas	(0) 1 4 8
17. Generally constipated (or straining during bowel movements)	0 (1) 4 8
18. Stool is small, hard, and dry	(0) 1 4 8
19. Pass mucus in your stool	(0) 1 4 8
20. Alternate between constipation and diarrhea	(0) 1 4 8
21. Rectal pain, itching, or cramping	(0) 1 4 8
22. No urge to have a bowel movement	(0) 1 4 8
23. Do you have an almost continual need to have a bowel movement?	(0) No (8) Yes
Total Points Part I, Section A	4

Section B

1. When massaging under your rib cage on your right side, there is pain, tenderness, or soreness | (0) 1 4 8
2. Abdominal pain worsens with deep breathing | (0) 1 4 8
3. Pain at night that may move to your back or right shoulder | (0) 1 4 8
4. Bitter fluid repeats after eating | (0) 1 4 8
5. Feel abdominal discomfort or nausea when eating rich, fatty, or fried foods | (0) 1 4 8
6. Throbbing temples or dull pain in forehead associated with eating | (0) 1 4 8
7. Unexplained itchy skin that's worse at night | 0 (1) 4 8
8. Stool color alternates from clay colored to normal brown | 0 (1) 4 8
9. General feeling of poor health | (0) 1 4 8
10. Aching muscles not due to exercise | (0) 1 4 8
11. Retain fluid and feel swollen around the abdominal area | (0) 1 4 8
12. Reddened skin, especially palms | (0) 1 4 8
13. Very strong body odor | (0) 1 4 8
14. Do you bruise easily? | (0)No (8)Yes
15. Is there a yellowish cast to eyes? | (0)No (8)Yes

Total Points Part I, Section B   2

Part II. Endocrine Health	
Section A	
1. Feel cold or chilled—hands, feet, or all over—for no apparent reason	0 (1) 4 8
2. Your upper eyelids look swollen	(0) 1 4 8
3. Muscles are weak, cramp, or tremble	(0) 1 4 8
4. You are forgetful and find it difficult to focus	0 (1) 4 8
5. Sensation of your heart beating slowly	0 (1) 4 8
6. Reaction time seems slowed down	0 (1) 4 8
7. Generally disinterested in sex because your desire is low	0 (1) 4 8
8. Feel slow-moving, sluggish	(0) 1 4 8
9. Constipation (or straining during a bowel movement)	0 (1) 4 8
10. Do you have swelling of the neck	(0) 1 4 8
11. Experience a depressed mood	0 (1) 4 8
12. Have you been diagnosed with elevated cholesterol?	(0) 1 4 8
13. Is your skin or hair dry or discolored?	(0)No (8)Yes
14. Have you noticed recently that your voice is deepening?	(0)No (8)Yes
15. Do you have thick, brittle nails?	(0)No (8)Yes
16. Have you gained weight for no apparent reason?	(0)No (8)Yes
17. Is the outer third of your eyebrow thinning or disappearing?	(0)No (8)Yes
18. Difficulties associated with menstrual cycle	(0)No (8)Yes
19. Have you had difficulty getting pregnant?	(0)No (8)Yes
Total Points Part II, Section A	7

Section B

1.	Lingering mild fatigue after exertion or stress	0 ①/4 8
2.	You get tired and exhaust easily	0 ①4 8
3.	Craving for salty foods	0 ①4 8
4.	Dizzy when rising or standing up from a kneeling position	⓪1 4 8
5.	Dark bluish or black circles under your eyes	⓪1 4 8
6.	Bouts of nausea with or without vomiting	⓪1 4 8
7.	Your body or part of your body feels tender, sore, sensitive to the touch, hot, or painful	⓪1 4 8
8.	Feel puffy and swollen all over your body	⓪1 4 8
9.	Carry extra weight around your abdomen	0 ①4 8
10.	Poor body composition (too much fat vs. lean tissue)	0 ①4 8
11.	Need caffeine to get you going in the morning	⓪1 4 8
12.	Your are forgetful and find it difficult to focus	⓪1 4 8
13.	Feeling emotionally flat or lacking zest for living	0 ①4 8
14.	Feel nervous or anxious	⓪1 4 8
15.	Generally disinterested in sex because your desire is low	0 ①4 8
16.	Do you have trouble falling asleep, or staying asleep?	(0)No (8)Yes
17.	Do you easily catch colds or infections?	(0)No (8)Yes
18.	Do wounds heal slowly?	(0)No (8)Yes
19.	Is your skin gradually tanning without exposure to sun?	(0)No (8)Yes
20.	Have you been diagnosed with high blood pressure?	(0)No (8)Yes
21.	Have you been diagnosed with elevated cholesterol?	(0)No (8)Yes
22.	Have you been diagnosed with high blood sugar?	(0)No (8)Yes

Total Points Part II, Section B   7   8

Part III. Sugar Regulation	
Section A	
When you miss meals or go without food for extended periods of time, do you experience any of the following symptoms?	
1. A sense of weakness	0 (1) 4 8
2. A sudden sense of anxiety when you get hungry	0 (1) 4 8
3. Tingling sensation in your hands	(0) 1 4 8
4. A sensation of your heart beating too quickly or forcefully	0 (1) 4 8
5. Shaky, jittery hands, trembling	(0) 1 4 8
6. Sudden profuse sweating or clammy skin	(0) 1 4 8
7. Wake up at night feeling restless	0 (1) 4 8
8. Nightmares possibly associated with going to bed on an empty stomach	(0) 1 4 8
9. Agitation, easily upset, nervous	(0) 1 4 8
10. Poor memory, forgetful	0 (1) 4 8
11. Confused or disoriented	(0) 1 4 8
12. Dizzy, faint	(0) 1 4 8
13. Cold or numb	(0) 1 4 8
14. Mild headaches or head pounding	(0) 1 4 8
15. Blurred vision or double vision	(0) 1 4 8
16. Feel clumsy and uncoordinated	(0) 1 4 8
Total Points Part III, Section A	5
Section B	
1. Frequent urination during the day and night	0 (1) 4 8
2. Unusual thirst, feeling like you can't drink enough water	(0) 1 4 8
3. Unusual hunger, eating all the time	(0) 1 4 8
4. Vision blurs	(0) 1 4 8
5. Feel itchy all over	0 (1) 4 8
6. Tingling or numbness in your feet	0 (1) 4 8
7. Sense of drowsiness, lethargy during the day not associated with missing meals or loss of sleep	0 (1) 4 8
8. Eating starchy foods causes you to gain weight or prevents you from losing weight	(0) 1 4 8
9. Wounds heal slowly	0 1 4 8
10. Do you notice a loss of hair on you legs?	(0)No (8)Yes
Total Points Part III, Section B	4 - 8

Part IV. Cardiovascular Health	
1. Feel jittery	(0) 1 4 8
2. First effort of the day causes pain, pressure, tightness, or heaviness around the chest	(0) 1 4 8
3. Exhaustion with minor exertion	0 (1) 4 8
4. Heavy sweating (no exertion, no hot flashes)	(0) 1 4 8
5. Difficulty catching breath, especially during exercise	0 (1) 4 8
6. Heart pounding or sensation of heart beating too quickly, too slowly, or irregularly	0 1 (4) 8
7. Swelling in feet, ankles, or legs comes and goes for no apparent reason	(0) 1 4 8
Total Points Part IV	
Part V. Mood	4
1. Family, friends, work, hobbies, or activities you hold dear are no longer of interest	(0) 1 4 8
2. Easily cry	0 (1) 4 8
3. Life looks entirely hopeless	(0) 1 4 8
4. You describe yourself as feeling miserable, sad, unhappy, or blue	0 (1) 4 8
5. You find it hard to make the best of difficult situations	0 (1) 4 8
6. Sleep problems, too much or too little sleep	0 1 (4) 8
7. Have there been changes in your appetite and weight?	(0)No (8)Yes
8. Lately have you noticed an inability to think clearly or concentrate?	(0)No (8)Yes
9. Do you have difficulty making decisions or clarifying and achieving your goals?	(0)No (8)Yes
Total Points Part V	7

Part VI. Immune Health	
1. Eyes water or tear	(0) 1 4 8
2. Discharge from the eyes or ears	0 (1) 4 8
3. Ears ache, itch, or feel congested or sore	(0) 1 4 8
4. Nose is continually congested	0 1 (4) 8
5. Nose runs	0 1 (4) 8
6. Clearing your throat	0 1 (4) 8
7. Feel a choking lump in your throat	(0) 1 4 8
8. Breathing difficulties	0 (1) 4 8
9. Chest discomfort or pain	(0) 1 4 8
10. Sudden breathing difficulties	0 (1) 4 8
11. Struggle with shortness of breath	0 (1) 4 8
12. Difficulty exhaling (breathing out)	0 (1) 4 8
13. Inability to breathe comfortably while lying down	(0) 1 4 8
14. Troubled with coughing or cough up lots of phlegm	0 1 (4) 8
15. Hear noisy rattling sounds when breathing in and out	(0) 1 4 8
16. Troubled with wheezing	(0) 1 4 8
17. Severe soaking sweats at night	(0) 1 4 8
18. Sleepy during the day	0 (1) 4 8
19. Difficulty concentrating	0 (1) 4 8
20. Do eyes, ears, nose, throat, and lung symptoms seem associated with specific foods such as dairy or wheat products?	(0)No (8)Yes
21. Sensitive to perfumes, cleaning products, mold, mildew, gas fumes, pollution, etc.?	(0)No (8)Yes
22. Have you been told you have chronic fatigue syndrome?	(0)No (8)Yes
23. Have you been told you have autoimmune disease?	(0)No (8)Yes
24. Are you prone to loud snoring?	(0)No (8)Yes
25. Do you experience nosebleeds?	(0)No (8)Yes
26. Do you suffer from severe colds?	(0)No (8)Yes
27. Do frequent colds keep you miserable all winter?	(0)No (8)Yes
28. Do flu symptoms last longer than five days?	(0)No (8)Yes
29. Do infections settle in your lungs?	(0)No (8)Yes
Total Points Part VI	20

Part VII. Musculoskeletal Health	
Section A	
1. Bones throughout your entire body ache or feel tender or sore	(0) 1 4 8
2. Localized bone pain	0 (1) 4 8
3. Upper or lower back pain	(0) 1 4 8
4. Pain when sitting down or walking	0 (1) 4 8
5. Stiffness in the morning when you wake up	0 (1) 4 8
6. Difficulty bending down and picking up things from the floor	0 (1) 4 8
7. Joint swelling, pain, or stiffness involving one or more areas	0 1 (4) 8
8. Joints hurt when moving or when carrying weight	0 (1) 4 8
9. Numbness, prickling, or tingling sensation, or pain in neck, shoulder, or arm	0 (1) 4 8
10. Muscles stiff, sore, tense, or achy	0 (1) 4 8
11. Muscle cramps or spasms (involuntary or after exertion or exercise)	(0) 1 4 8
12. Specific points on body feel sore when pressed	0 (1) 4 8
13. Feel unrefreshed upon awakening	0 (1) 4 8
14. Headaches	(0) 1 4 8
15. Muscle twitch or tremor in the eyelids, thumb, calf muscle	0 (1) 4 8
16. Is it difficult to reach up and get a five-pound object like a bag of flour from just above your head?	(0)No (8)Yes
17. Do you injure, strain, or sprain easily?	(0)No (8)Yes
Total Points Part VII	13

Part VIII. Female Health	
Section A *(Menopausal women skip to Section B)* *Do you persistently experience any of these symptoms within three days to two weeks prior to menstruation?*	
1. Profuse heavy bleeding during periods	0 1 4 8
2. Menstrual blood contains clots and tissue	0 1 4 8
3. Bleeding between periods can occur at any time	0 1 4 8
4. Anxious, irritable, easy to anger, or restless	(0)No (8)Yes
5. Numbness or tingling in hands and feet	(0)No (8)Yes
6. Abdominal bloating, swollen feeling (e.g., in feet)	(0)No (8)Yes
7. Temporary weight gain	(0)No (8)Yes
8. Breast tenderness, swelling	(0)No (8)Yes
9. Appearance of breast lumps	(0)No (8)Yes
10. Discharge from nipples	(0)No (8)Yes
11. Nausea or vomiting	(0)No (8)Yes
12. Diarrhea or constipation	(0)No (8)Yes
13. Aches and pains (back, joints, etc.)	(0)No (8)Yes
14. Craving for sweets	(0)No (8)Yes
15. Increased appetite or binge eating	(0)No (8)Yes
16. Headaches	(0)No (8)Yes
17. Being easily overwhelmed, shaky or clumsy	(0)No (8)Yes
18. Dizziness or fainting	(0)No (8)Yes
19. Overwhelmed with feelings of sadness and worthlessness	(0)No (8)Yes
20. Difficulty sleeping or falling asleep	(0)No (8)Yes
Total Points Part VIII, Section A	

Section B

1. Vaginal dryness		0 1 4 8
2. Sexual intercourse is uncomfortable		0 1 4 8
3. Interest in having sex is low		0 1 4 8
4. Difficulty with orgasm		0 1 4 8
5. Vaginal bleeding after sexual intercourse		0 1 4 8
6. Sense of well-being fluctuates throughout the day for no apparent reason		0 1 4 8
7. Sudden hot flashes		0 1 4 8
8. Spontaneous sweating		0 1 4 8
9. Chills		0 1 4 8
10. Cold hands and feet		0 1 4 8
11. Heart beats rapidly or feels like it is fluttering		0 1 4 8
12. Numbness, tingling, or prickling sensations		0 1 4 8
13. Dizziness		0 1 4 8
14. Mental fogginess, forgetful or distracted		0 1 4 8
15. Inability to concentrate		0 1 4 8
16. Depression, anxiety, nervousness, or irritability		0 1 4 8
17. Difficulty sleeping		0 1 4 8
18. Conscious of new feelings of anger and frustration		0 1 4 8
19. Skin, hair, or eyes feel dry		0 1 4 8

Total Points Part VIII, Section B

Part IX. Sleep	
1. Difficulty falling asleep or staying asleep	0 1 ④ 8
2. Wake early and cannot fall back asleep	0 1 ④ 8
3. A significant amount of emotional stress	0 ① 4 8
4. Breathing problems	0 ① 4 8
5. Take prescription medication	0 1 ④ 8
6. Use of recreational drugs, alcohol, or stimulants, including coffee, tea, energy drinks, colas, or chocolate	0 1 ④ 8
7. Snore heavily	0 ① 4 8
8. Waken due to a sensation of choking	⓪ 1 4 8
9. Restless sleep	0 ① 4 8
10. Wake with a morning headache	⓪ 1 4 8
11. Irresistible urge to move legs	0 ① 4 8
12. Legs move during sleep	0 ① 4 8
13. Unpleasant crawling sensation inside calves when lying down	0 ① 4 8
14. Are you currently withdrawing from the use of drugs?	(0)No (8)Yes
15. Have you been told that you suffer from chronic kidney or liver problems?	(0)No (8)Yes
16. Are you pregnant?	(0)No (8)Yes
17. Have you been told you are anemic?	(0)No (8)Yes
18. Do you frequently travel across two or more time zones or work irregular hours?	(0)No (8)Yes
19. Have you recently stopped taking medication to help you sleep?	(0)No (8)Yes
20. Do you have chronic pain?	(0)No (8)Yes
21. Are you obese and sleep on your back?	(0)No (8)Yes
Total Points Part IX	2 1

Part X. Environmental Health	
1. Use pesticides, herbicides, or fungicides at home, work or during hobbies	0 (1) 4 8
2. Shower or bathe in chlorinated water	0 (1) 4 8
3. Drink from or store food in plastic containers	0 (1) 4 8
4. Exposed to chemical toxins at home, work or during hobbies	0 (1) 4 8
5. Consume processed foods that contain artificial colors, additives, preservatives	0 (1) 4 8
6. Use non-natural or non-organic body and home care products including cleaners, soaps, cream, toothpaste, hair care products, make-up, perfumes etc.	0 (1) 4 8
7. Wear clothing that is dry cleaned	(0) 1 4 8
8. Mold or mildew in your home or work environment	(0) 1 4 8
9. Poorer tolerance to environmental toxins than most of those around you	(0) 1 4 8
10. Sensitive to perfumes, cleaning products, mold, mildew, gas fumes, pollution, etc.	(0) 1 4 8
11. Do you drink unfiltered, chlorinated, or fluorinated water?	(0)No (8)Yes
12. In the past 5 years have you lived or worked in a new building?	(0)No (8)Yes
13. Do you eat unwashed fruits and vegetables?	(0)No (8)Yes
14. Do you regularly microwave items in plastic containers?	(0)No (8)Yes
15. Do you cook in aluminum pots and pans or consume canned foods?	(0)No (8)Yes
16. Do you use antiperspirants that contain aluminum?	(0)No (8)Yes
17. Do you or have you had silver fillings in your teeth?	(0)No (8)Yes
18. Have you been diagnosed with any of the following disorders; migraine headaches, autoimmune disorders, depression, ADHD, asthma, chronic fatigue syndrome, fibromyalgia, cancer, multiple chemical sensitivity, Parkinson's disease, and Alzheimer's disease?	(0)No (8)Yes
19. Have you ever or do you currently live with a smoker or smoke yourself?	(0)No (8)Yes
20. Do you or have you lived or worked in an area that is highly polluted?	(0)No (8)Yes
Total Points Part X	
Total Points All Sections	6 56

The Many Faces of Fatigue

Note

I have used two main sources in verifying this information, *The Merck Manual* and the *Textbook of Natural Medicine*.

Digestive Health

Part I, Section A

Maldigestion

An underactive digestive system does not produce enough stomach acid or digestive enzymes for the adequate digestion of food. Bile secretion, Vitamin B_{12} absorption, and the enzymes responsible for the digestion of protein are activated by stomach acid. If stomach acid is insufficient, it results in inadequate breakdown of food, most notably protein and fat. Insufficient stomach acid also promotes overgrowth of bacteria and toxin formation in the intestines.

Failure to practice the principles of healthy living is the most common underlying cause, particularly a diet consistently high in meat (especially red meat), dairy products, refined, processed, and fast foods. Stomach acid production decreases with age, so the condition is more common in people over forty.

Conditions associated with low stomach acid include: small bowel intestinal overgrowth, yeast overgrowth, H. pylori infection, Addison's disease, asthma, diabetes, eczema, psoriasis, autoimmune disorders, hypothyroidism, chronic hives, osteoporosis, pernicious anemia, rheumatoid arthritis, lupus, and gallbladder disease.

Signs and Symptoms

Belching, indigestion, and passing gas (especially after meals); diarrhea or constipation; poor absorption of protein and minerals; anemia; multiple food allergies; nausea after taking supplements; itching around the rectum; chronic intestinal parasites; undigested food in the stool; fatigue; weak, peeling, or cracked fingernails; dilated blood vessels in the cheeks and nose; and acne.

Malabsorption

Malabsorption, simply put, means poor absorption of food by the intestinal cells. It is most often due to inadequate breakdown of fats, proteins, and carbohydrates, resulting in poor absorption and transport of digested food by-products. This results in their excessive excretion in the stool, producing both digestive symptoms and nutritional deficiencies.

Signs and Symptoms

Gas; abdominal distension and bloating; diarrhea; foul-smelling, pale, bulky, or greasy stools; fatigue; weight loss; and symptoms of nutritional and vitamin or mineral deficiencies.

Maldigestion and Malabsorption

Confirmatory Testing

- History—Vitamin and mineral nutrient screening questionnaire.
- Blood Studies—Screen for anemia, vitamin/nutrient deficiencies, albumin, cholesterol, H. pylori, and bleed time.
- Gastric Acid Analyses—Heidelberg gastric analysis measures the ability of the stomach to secrete acid. Hydrochloric acid challenge uses oral supplementation used to estimate functional stomach acid levels.
- Urine Studies—The lactulose-mannitol oral challenge measures mannitol and lactulose following an oral challenge. The Obermeyer, or urinary indican, test provides an index of the efficiency of protein digestion. The pancreolauryl test measures pancreatic function following an oral challenge.
- Blood and Urine Studies—D-xylose absorption test measures D-xylose after an oral challenge.
- Stool Studies—Comprehensive digestive stool analysis evaluates digestion, intestinal function, intestinal environment, and absorption. Near-infrared reflectance analysis tests the stool for fat, nitrogen, and carbohydrates. Measure fecal fat in the stool over seventy-two hours. Fecal Elastase-1 is an indirect measure of pancreatic function.

Anemia

When cells in the kidney detect low oxygen levels in the blood, they signal the production of more red blood cells. This production requires adequate supplies of iron, Vitamin B_{12}, and folate. If these stores are not adequate due to poor intake, absorption, or assimilation of the necessary building blocks, anemia results. Iron-deficiency anemia is the most common type, especially among women and the elderly.

Common causes include: vegetarianism, insufficient stomach acid, bleeding from the digestive tract, malabsorption, heavy menstrual periods, and greater than one past pregnancy.

Signs and Symptoms

Fatigue and shortness of breath with slight exertion, irritability, pale complexion, weakness, drowsiness, vertigo, headache, ringing in the ears, spots before the eyes, loss of sex drive, and scanty menstruation.

Confirmatory Testing

- Blood Studies—Complete blood count, ferritin, vitamin B_{12}, and folate levels.
- Stool Studies—Screen for presence of blood.
- Gastric Acid Analyses—Heidelberg gastric analysis measures the ability of the stomach to secrete acid. Hydrochloric acid challenge uses oral supplementation used to estimate functional stomach acid levels.

Small Intestinal Bowel Overgrowth

In small intestinal bowel overgrowth, a greater than optimal concentration of bacteria exists in the small intestine. Alterations in normal functioning of the digestive system promote bacterial overgrowth.

Predisposing factors include: low stomach acid, underactive digestive system, intestinal stasis and chronic constipation, maldigestion, malabsorption, leaky gut syndrome, use of acid blocking medications, prior intestinal surgery, carbohydrate intolerance, damaged ileocecal valve, and an underactive immune system.

It is associated with diabetes, scleroderma, Crohn's disease, aging, irritable bowel syndrome, fibromyalgia, chronic fatigue syndrome, diverticulosis, and celiac disease.

Signs and Symptoms

Gas, bloating, abdominal cramping and diarrhea (usually after eating), lactose intolerance, symptoms of protein and fat malabsorption, deficiencies in fat-soluble vitamins, bone loss, Vitamin B_{12} deficient anemia, *fatigue,* and weight loss.

Confirmatory Testing

- Breath Tests—Measure hydrogen or methane following ingestion of a carbohydrate.
- Urine Studies—Obermeyer test provides an index of the efficiency of protein digestion.
- Endoscopy—To culture the small bowel.
- Stool Analysis—Comprehensive digestive stool analysis evaluates digestion, intestinal function, intestinal environment, and absorption, and can help distinguish between small intestinal bacterial overgrowth, leaky gut syndrome, and yeast overgrowth.

Yeast Overgrowth (Candidiasis)

A normal resident of the digestive and vaginal tracts, *Candida albicans*, is a yeast fungus that has received a lot of attention to date. When it grows out of control, our delicate balance of microorganisms is upset.

Although necessary at times, chronic use of antibiotics is the greatest predisposing factor to yeast overgrowth. Antibiotics are designed to kill bad bacteria that cause disease, but unfortunately they are not completely selective. They also kill the good bacteria that are essential for intestinal and immune health.

Common causes, other than antibiotic use, include: failure to practice the principles of healthy living, stress, maldigestion, underactive immune system, pregnancy, and use of steroids or oral birth control.

Signs and Symptoms

Chronic fatigue, a generalized feeling of ill health, headaches, depression, inability to concentrate, decreased sex drive, bloating, gas, intestinal cramps, rectal itching, constipation or diarrhea, sensitivity to foods and chemicals, allergies, difficulty in losing weight, yeast and bladder infections, insatiable hunger, joint pain, poor immune function, hormonal disturbance, eczema, psoriasis, and skin rashes, as well as cravings for refined carbohydrates, sugar, or yeast.

Confirmatory Testing

- History—Diagnosis is best made by evaluation of a patient's history and clinical picture. Candida screening questionnaire.
- Blood Studies—Candida antibody test measures the level of antibodies to *Candida albicans* (*C. albicans*) or the level of antigens in the blood.

Candisphere enzyme immuno-assay test measures enzymes from the cytoplasm of the *C. albicans* cell.

- Urine Studies—Organic acid urine test measures the metabolites formed by *C. albicans* in the body. The Obermeyer test provides an index of the efficiency of protein digestion.

- Stool Culture—Quantitative Candida stool culture measures the amount of *C. albicans* in the stool. Comprehensive digestive stool analysis evaluates digestion, intestinal function, intestinal environment, and absorption. It can help distinguish between small intestinal bacterial overgrowth, leaky gut syndrome, and *C. albicans* overgrowth.

Leaky Gut Syndrome (Intestinal Permeability)

In leaky gut syndrome, there is damage to the integrity of the intestinal lining, thus diminishing its ability to screen unwanted food particles, toxins, and pathogens. When proteins are not adequately digested, they are absorbed through a leaky gut and stimulate the immune system. Over time it may contribute to allergies, digestive disorders, and arthritic or autoimmune disorders.

Predisposing factors include: maldigestion, malabsorption, and bacterial or yeast overgrowth.

It is associated with acne, alcoholism, celiac disease, chronic fatigue syndrome, Crohn's disease, cystic fibrosis, eczema and psoriasis, food allergies, hyperactivity, irritable bowel syndrome, sluggish liver, multiple chemical sensitivities, pancreatic insufficiency, rheumatoid arthritis, lupus, weight gain, eczema, and psoriasis.

Signs and Symptoms

Any of the signs and symptoms of maldigestion, malabsorption, small intestinal bowel and yeast overgrowth, sluggish liver, and allergies.

Confirmatory Testing

- Urine Studies—Lactulose-mannitol challenge is used to measure intestinal permeability. It measures mannitol and lactulose after an oral challenge.

- Stool Studies—Comprehensive digestive stool analysis evaluates digestion, intestinal function, intestinal environment, and absorption. Helps distinguish between small intestinal bacterial overgrowth, leaky gut syndrome, and yeast overgrowth.

- Screening—Any of the appropriate tests for maldigestion, malabsorption, and small intestinal bowel and yeast overgrowth can be ordered, based on individual history and presenting signs and symptoms.

Inflammatory Bowel Disease (Crohn's and Ulcerative Colitis)

Inflammatory bowel disease is characterized by chronic inflammation at various sites in the digestive tract. It is divided into two major categories, Crohn's disease and ulcerative colitis.

Crohn's disease is characterized by inflammation and abscess formation leading to patchy areas of ulcerated tissue. It involves the entire thickness of the intestinal wall, most commonly affecting the far end of the small intestine and the large intestine.

Ulcerative colitis is characterized by inflammation and ulceration of the large intestine and bloody diarrhea. It commonly begins in the rectum extending upwards, eventually involving the entire large intestine. It is associated with arthritis and increased risk of colon cancer.

Signs and Symptoms

Usually intermittent, signs and symptoms include: cramping, diarrhea; abdominal pain and distension; urgency to defecate; blood, pus, or mucus in the stools; constipation; vomiting; a general sense of feeling ill; fever; loss of appetite; fatigue; weight loss; and malnutrition.

Confirmatory Testing

- Physical Exam of Abdomen
- Blood Studies—Measure the markers of inflammation. Screen for anemia, leukocytosis, hypoalbuminemia, electrolyte abnormalities, and liver function.
- X-rays—Abdominal x-rays show abnormalities associated with Crohn's disease and the upper extent of ulcerative colitis. Barium enema x-ray shows abnormalities associated with the large intestine.
- Endoscopic Examination—Endoscopy, colonoscopy, or sigmoidoscopy allow for visualization and biopsy.
- Stool Studies—Evaluate presence of white blood cells, ova and parasites, pH, fat, and electrolytes. Comprehensive digestive stool analysis evaluates digestion, intestinal function, intestinal environment, and absorption and

can help distinguish other digestive disorders from inflammatory bowel disease.

Part I, Section B

Sluggish Liver

One of the liver's many jobs is to filter the blood, removing or neutralizing toxins. Another is to produce bile for the digestion of fats. When the liver is overburdened by toxin exposure or excessive intake of dietary fat, it becomes what has been loosely termed a sluggish liver. A sluggish liver results in the compromise of several liver functions, including detoxification, bile production, the digestion of fats, assimilation of fat-soluble nutrients, sterilization of microorganisms in the digestive tract, intestinal lubrication, and hormone management.

Failure to practice the principles of healthy living is the most common underlying cause, in addition to chronic, high exposure to toxins.

A sluggish liver is associated with high levels of free radicals, obesity, diabetes, gallstones, premenstrual syndrome, multiple chemical sensitivity, skin conditions such as eczema and psoriasis, and chronic use of over-the-counter and prescription medication.

Signs and Symptoms

Generalized feeling of ill health, depressed mood, headaches, fatigue, digestive disturbances, allergies, chemical sensitivity, and constipation.

Confirmatory Testing

- Blood Studies—Standard liver function tests are only useful if there is significant damage to liver which is uncommon in this stage of dysfunction. Bile acid assay measures liver function.

- Urine and Saliva Studies—Comprehensive liver detoxification profile measures the liver's detoxification ability following an oral challenge.

Endocrine Health

Part II, Section A

Underactive Thyroid (Hypothyroidism)

An underactive thyroid is characterized by a deficiency of thyroid hormone resulting in changes in temperature regulation and metabolism. There are two kinds of underactive thyroid, primary and secondary. In primary hypothyroidism, the thyroid itself is responsible; in secondary hypothyroidism, the pituitary gland is responsible for the low level of thyroid hormone.

It is often failure to practice the principles of healthy living that eventually impacts the thyroid, long after other systems have been affected. Autoimmune disease, where your own body attacks itself, and iodine deficiency are other possible causes, but iodine deficiency is rare in countries where iodized table salt is used.

Primary Hypothyroidism (most common)

Signs and Symptoms

Fatigue; forgetfulness; difficulty losing weight; elevated cholesterol; constipation; menstrual problems; headache; recurrent infections; depressed mood; dry, rough, and scaly skin; sensitivity to cold; cold hands and feet; hair loss with coarse, dry, brittle hair; thin, brittle nails with transverse grooves; tingling sensations in the hands and feet; muscle pain or weakness; joint stiffness and pain; hoarse voice; and orange discoloration on palms of hand and soles of feet.

Secondary Hypothyroidism (rare)

Signs and Symptoms

History of no menstruation, dry skin and hair, loss of skin color, slightly enlarged tongue, decreased breast fullness, low blood pressure, low blood sugar, and a small heart.

Confirmatory Testing

- Physical Examination—Palpation of the thyroid gland, Achilles tendon reflex, and basal body temperature measurements.

- Blood Studies—Measure thyroid stimulating hormone, thyroid hormone, thyroid binding globulin. Unfortunately, routine blood tests are not always sensitive enough to detect a mildly underactive thyroid. The patient presents with clinical signs and symptoms of an underactive thyroid, but blood studies reveal normal levels of circulating thyroid hormone. For a more complete analysis of thyroid function, measurement of freeT4, freeT3 and rT3 can be performed. Other tests include the thyroid releasing hormone test to differentiate between primary and secondary types, autoimmune testing to detect autoimmune thyroid disease, and screening for elevated cholesterol and anemia, as they are commonly associated with an underactive thyroid.

Part II, Section B

Adrenal Dysfunction (General Adaptation Syndrome)

As discussed earlier, the adrenal glands are primarily responsible for our body's response to stress, whether the stress is physical, mental, emotional, or spiritual. General adaptation syndrome (GAS) specifically affects our adrenal glands and consists of three phases: alarm, resistance, and exhaustion. When you first encounter stress, you will feel stressed and wired; this is the alarm phase of GAS. If the stress persists, you will become stressed and tired; this is the resistance phase of GAS. If the stress is still not relieved, you will feel stressed and burnt out, moving towards the exhaustion phase. The associated feeling of fatigue increases the desire to use stimulants, medication, and alcohol, all of which worsen the condition. Prolonged stress and failure to practice the principles of healthy living are the most common underlying causes.

Signs and Symptoms

Anxiety, fatigue, exhaustion, dizziness, and drop in blood pressure upon standing, disturbed sleep, headache, emotional alterations and depression, dark coloration of skin, digestive complaints, disturbance in metabolism of food, difficulty regulating blood sugar, difficulty losing weight, and weight gain.

Confirmatory Testing

- History—Significant or prolonged stress. Stress inventory questionnaire.
- Physical Exam—Orthostatic blood pressure.
- Blood Studies—Measure substances related to adrenal function, including DHEA, cortisol, and hormones.
- Salivary Studies—Measure DHEA and cortisol levels.
- Urine Studies—Koenisburg test is an indirect measurement of sodium excretion.

Obesity

Obesity is a term used to describe poor body composition or an excessive amount of fat. Body composition is the ratio of fat to lean tissue in the body. To date, most people have relied on the mirror, the scale, and height/weight charts to estimate their body composition. When you step on the scale, however, that number does nothing to tell you how much fat you have or its distribution on your body.

Failure to practice the principles of healthy living is the most common underlying cause.

Obesity is associated with increased risk of belly fat, diabetes, metabolic syndrome, cardiovascular disease, stroke, cancer, and the inflammatory diseases.

Belly fat is the term used to describe the deposition of fat around the abdominal organs, resembling an apple shape. Excess belly fat increases generalized inflammation in the body, damaging joints, blood vessels, and the immune system. Belly fat triggers a series of events that, if left untreated, result in elevated cholesterol, type 2 diabetes, and cardiovascular disease.

Signs and Symptoms

Weight gain, poor body composition, and generalized fatigue.

Confirmatory Testing

- Body Mass Index (BMI)—The BMI is a widely used index of desirable weight for adults thought to correlate well with body composition and in turn disease risk. To calculate your BMI, you may use one of the following equations,

    BMI = Weight (lb) x 703 divided by Height (in)^2

    Metric BMI = Weight (kg) divided by Height (m)^2

    A BMI from 19–24 is considered normal, over 25 is considered overweight, over 30 is considered obese, and over 40 is considered extremely obese. In terms of body composition, obesity is defined as a body fat percentage greater than 30 percent for women and 25 percent for men. Since risk of disease increases incrementally with each percent of fat above optimal, it is recommended that body fat be maintained in the optimal range. Currently, optimal ranges are 10–15 percent for men and 15–20 percent for women. Remember that it is considered unhealthy for women to maintain a total body fat percentage less than 10 percent and for men, less than 5 percent.

- Analysis of Skinfold Thickness—Measures skinfold thickness using a skinfold caliper at one or more sites on the body.

- Bioelectrical Impedance Analysis (BIA)—BIA provides an estimate of the percentage of body fat by sending an electrical current through the body.

- Hydrostatic Weighing—Measures the weight of the body both in and out of water.

Metabolic Syndrome

Metabolic syndrome, also known as syndrome X and as metabolic cardiovascular risk syndrome, is characterized by a combination of three or more of the following: abdominal obesity, high blood sugar, elevated triglycerides, elevated cholesterol, and high blood pressure.

Failure to practice the principles of healthy living is the most common underlying cause.

Signs and Symptoms

Elevated cholesterol, high blood pressure, excess belly fat, and any symptoms previously listed for high blood sugar and obesity.

Confirmatory Testing

- Waist Circumference or Waist-to-Hip Ratio—Circumference of the waist divided by circumference of the hips.

- Blood Studies—Measure fasting total cholesterol, triglycerides, high density lipoproteins, and low density lipoproteins. Other tests measure insulin, fasting glucose, or glucose following ingestion of a meal.

- Skin Test—Measures skin tissue cholesterol content.

- Blood Pressure—Measured in mmHg:

	Systolic		Diastolic
Optimal	< 120	and	< 80
Prehypertension	120–139	or	80–89
Stage 1 hypertension	140–159	or	90–99
Stage 2 hypertension	≥ 160	or	≥100

Sugar Regulation

Part III, Section A

Low Blood Sugar (Hypoglycemia)

There are two separate categories of abnormally low blood sugar: reactive and fasting. Reactive hypoglycemia is the most common and is characterized by the development of the symptoms of low blood sugar three to five hours after a meal, especially after a meal that is rich in carbohydrates, which stimulates excess insulin production. It may precede the onset of type 2 diabetes. Fasting hypoglycemia is rare and is characterized by the development of the symptoms of low blood sugar after a period of prolonged fasting or prolonged strenuous exercise.

Failure to practice the principles of healthy living is the most common underlying cause, most notably the overconsumption of refined carbohydrates (especially sugar).

Signs and Symptoms

Light-headedness, headache, hunger, nausea, shakiness, weakness, sweating, palpitations, mood swings, tingling sensations, confusion, irritability, fatigue, and visual disturbances.

Confirmatory Testing

- Blood Studies—Measure insulin, random glucose, fasting glucose, or glucose after ingestion of a meal. Glucose tolerance test measures blood glucose after an oral challenge. Glucose-insulin tolerance test measures blood glucose and insulin after an oral challenge. Glycosylated hemoglobin indirectly measures blood sugar levels over the past three months.

Part III, Section B

High Blood Sugar (Diabetes)

If blood sugar remains elevated, insulin levels rise in order to bring blood sugar back into a healthy range. If blood sugar levels remain elevated despite adequate insulin secretion, more insulin is released in an attempt to decrease these levels. Eventually the cells stop listening to insulin signaling, which is termed insulin insensitivity, and blood sugar levels continue to rise. Chronically elevated blood sugar levels ultimately result in a condition known as type 2 diabetes.

Failure to practice the principles of healthy living is the most common underlying cause, most notably excessive intake of refined carbohydrates (especially sugar).

Signs and Symptoms

Symptoms are often mild and can go unnoticed. It is commonly detected on routine testing; however, weight gain around the midsection is one of the first signs to arise. More severe symptoms include: fatigue, frequent urination, excessive thirst, excessive hunger, blurred vision, slowed healing, frequent infections, and eventually cardiovascular disease.

Confirmatory Testing

- History—Symptoms appear three to five hours after eating or prolonged periods of fasting and are alleviated after a meal.
- Blood Studies—Blood glucose levels measured while symptoms are present. Glucose tolerance test measures blood glucose after an oral challenge of glucose. Glucose-insulin tolerance test measures blood glucose and insulin after an oral challenge of glucose. Hypoglycemic Index is a calculation of the severity of low blood sugar levels using blood glucose measurements.

Cardiovascular Health

Part IV

Coronary Artery Disease

Coronary artery disease involves a restriction of blood flow through the arteries that supply the heart. The most common cause of this restriction is called plaque. Plaque is an accumulation and swelling in the artery walls containing cholesterol, fatty acids, calcium, and fibrous tissue. Risk factors include high cholesterol, type 2 diabetes, obesity, belly fat, high blood pressure, an underactive thyroid, and the inflammatory diseases.

Failure to practice the principles of healthy living is the most common underlying cause.

Signs and Symptoms

Symptoms are often mild and can go unnoticed due to silent episodes of restricted blood flow. Early signs: exhaustion with only minor exertion; difficulty catching breath (especially during exercise); the sensation of pain, pressure, tightness, or heaviness around the chest; and heavy sweating (unrelated to exertion or hot flashes).

Confirmatory Testing

- History
- Electrocardiogram—Measures the activity of the heart.
- Stress Testing—Measures the response of the heart to exertion.
- Diagnostic Imaging—Coronary angiography visualizes the plaques.

Mood

Part V

Depressed Mood (Dysthymia)

Low-level depressive symptoms are classified as the mood disorder dysthymia. Symptoms often begin subtly during adolescence and follow a low-grade, on-and-off pattern over many years.

People may have a genetic predisposition that is triggered by failure to practice the principles of healthy living, psychosocial factors, altered brain neurotransmitter levels, or hormonal function.

Signs and Symptoms

Fatigue, feeling habitually gloomy or pessimistic, incapable of having fun, passivity, introversion, being skeptical or critical of self and others, feeling not good enough, and focusing on failure and negative events.

Confirmatory Testing

- History—Experiencing the above symptoms for greater than or equal to two years.
- Blood Studies—Measure DHEA, cortisol, and serotonin levels.
- Saliva Studies—Measure DHEA and cortisol levels.
- Specific Laboratory Tests—Tests to rule out conditions responsible for the depressive mood are ordered based on individual history and presenting signs and symptoms.

Immune Health

Part VI

Underactive Immune System

An underactive immune system can occur, specifically, in the digestive system, which houses approximately 60 percent of your immune system, and more generally, in the body. It predisposes to frequent and chronic infections and illness. In addition to fighting infection, the immune system is responsible for keeping precancerous cells under control. When the immune system is impaired, cancerous cells can prosper and infections take longer to resolve. And when infections linger so does fatigue.

Signs and Symptoms

Chronic or frequent infections of the ears, nose, throat, lungs, or bladder; cold sores, boils, and sties; chronic swelling of the lymph glands; poor wound healing; fatigue; and flare-ups of psoriasis, eczema, and oral or genital herpes.

Confirmatory Testing

- History—Frequent and chronic infections. Questionnaire to screen for underactive immune function.
- Blood Studies—Measure immune cell number and function.

Allergies

Allergies are any exaggerated immune response to a foreign substance. True allergies are recognized by the immediate onset of hives, swelling of the throat and tongue, and airway closure. Sensitivities are reactions that cause more subtle symptoms rather than full-blown allergic symptoms. As already discussed, a leaky gut is thought to be a causative factor in developing an overactive immune system and is associated with almost all types of allergies.

Conditions associated with allergies include: migraines, cardiovascular disease, all diseases whose names end in "-itis," autoimmune disease, bed-wetting, ear infections, gallbladder disease, childhood hyperactivity, low blood pressure, low blood sugar, glaucoma, celiac disease, asthma, chronic bronchitis, ulcers, sinusitis, depression, insomnia, skin conditions, menstrual abnormalities, Alzheimer's disease, cancer, diabetes, and obesity.

Common allergens include: wheat, dairy products (including milk and cheese), chocolate, citrus fruits, coffee, corn, peanuts and tree nuts, pesticide residues on food, refined sugars, soy, tomatoes, eggs, food additives, and yeast.

Signs and Symptoms

Chronic and frequent infections; canker sores; digestive complaints, bladder problems, or impaired kidney function; emotional dysfunction and mental changes; difficulty sleeping, fatigue, or joint pain; acne, skin rash; irregular heart beat; headache; itchy eyes, nose, throat or skin; runny nose, sneezing, nasal congestion, wheezing, or swelling; shortness of breath; and seizure.

Confirmatory Testing

- History—Patient history is generally more reliable than testing or screening alone.

- Oral Challenge Testing—Patient is placed on hypoallergenic diet, then suspected foods are reintroduced monitoring response.

- Pulse Testing—Monitors immediate response to an oral challenge.

- Conventional Skin Testing—Measures reaction to potential offending agents. Not considered very accurate for diagnosing allergic asthma or food allergy.

- Blood Studies—Measures cells that are elevated in allergy. The standard RAST test measures immediate reactions to potential offending substances but is not sensitive to delayed reactions. A more complete version of this test measures both immediate and delayed reactions. ELISA test measures antibodies to food additives, heavy metals, chemicals, and environmental pollutants. SAGE testing measures complement (part of the immune system) and delayed reactions to potential offending substances.

- Secretion Analysis—Secretory IgA measures feces or saliva for the presence of immune cells. Evaluates secretions from the eyes, nose and lungs for presence of immune cells.

- Screening—Any of the tests previously listed for maldigestion, malabsorption, and small intestinal bowel and yeast overgrowth, or leaky gut can be ordered, based on individual history and presenting signs and symptoms.

Autoimmune Disorders

In autoimmune disorders, the immune system wages war on the cells of its own body, resulting in inflammation and injury. Autoimmune disorders are associated with fatigue, inflammatory disorders, food allergies, and leaky gut syndrome.

Examples of autoimmune disorders include: multiple sclerosis, Grave's disease, Hashimoto's thyroiditis, chronic fatigue syndrome, scleroderma, Raynaud's disease, lupus, myasthenia gravis, Sjögren's syndrome, rheumatoid arthritis, ulcerative colitis, polymyalgia rheumatica, fibromyalgia, and prostatitis.

Signs and Symptoms and *Confirmatory Testing*

Each condition has its own clinical history, physical exam findings, and confirmatory testing, which are too numerous to list here.

Chronic Fatigue Syndrome

Chronic fatigue syndrome, also known as chronic fatigue or immune dysfunction syndrome, involves constant, severe, debilitating, and unexplained fatigue that is not relieved by rest.

Signs and Symptoms

Recurrent fatigue, sore throat, low-grade fever, lymph node swelling, headache, muscle and joint pain, intestinal discomfort, emotional distress, depression, difficulty focusing, and underactive immune function.

Confirmatory Testing

- Centers for Disease Control and Prevention Diagnostic Criteria—New onset of fatigue lasting more than six months with a 50 percent reduction in activity and concurrent exclusion of other diagnoses. Presence of either eight of the following symptoms or six of the symptoms and two of the three signs listed below.
  Symptoms: mild fever, recurrent sore throat, painful lymph nodes, muscle weakness, muscle pain, prolonged fatigue after exercise, recurrent headache, migratory joint pain, neurological or psychological complaints (sensitivity to bright light, forgetfulness, confusion, inability to concentrate, excessive irritability, depression), sleep disturbance (excessive sleep or inability to sleep), and sudden onset of symptom complex. **Signs**: low-grade fever, inflammation of the back of the throat without presence of discharge, and palpable or tender lymph nodes.

- History—Detailed medical history reviewing all of the systems of the body.

- Specific Laboratory Tests—Tests to rule out other diseases or to confirm suspicions are ordered, based on individual history and presenting signs and symptoms.

Musculoskeletal Health

Part VII

Chronic Inflammation and Oxidative Stress

The immune system responds to infection, injury, toxic exposures, allergens, and stress with a generalized process called inflammation. It is normally a protective process; however, if the underlying cause of inflammation is not resolved, it becomes chronic, damaging the joints, blood vessels, and immune system. In chronic inflammation, an imbalance occurs between the substances that promote inflammation and the substances that counteract it. Inflammation in turn produces free radicals, and free radicals are commonly associated with chronic disease and aging.

Oxygen is essential to sustain life, but if the by-products of its utilization, called free radicals, are not neutralized by antioxidants, they will trigger a cascade of events that damage protein, fats, cholesterol, and DNA. This tissue damage is thought to be responsible for premature aging. Free radical production is normal, and when it is balanced by adequate amounts of antioxidants, it does not cause disease. But if inflammation produces free radicals and those free radicals in turn initiate the inflammatory process, a negative cycle is initiated.

Causes of free radicals include: failure to practice the principles of healthy living, pollution, excessive exercise, infections, pesticides, radiation, exposure to sunlight, stress, excess fat tissue, toxins, and inflammation.

Excess free radical production is associated with Alzheimer's and Parkinson's disease, macular degeneration, neurological dysfunction, obesity, cancer, cardiovascular disease, diabetes, and arthritis.

Signs and Symptoms

Local signs of inflammation include: pain, redness, heat, swelling, and loss of function. Inflammation is involved with any condition ending in "-itis" as well as conditions such as chronic pain, belly fat, elevated cholesterol, diabetes, obesity, cardiovascular disease, allergies, eczema and psoriasis, Alzheimer's disease, cancer, and neurological and autoimmune disorders. Fatigue is a common symptom of both chronic pain and inflammation.

Confirmatory Testing

- Blood Studies—Measure the markers of inflammation.
- Specific Laboratory Tests—As appropriate to confirm suspicions based on individual history and presenting signs and symptoms.
- Blood and Urine Studies—Measure antioxidant levels.

Fibromyalgia

Fibromyalgia is characterized by at least three months of chronic widespread pain involving the spinal region, left/right as well as upper and lower parts of body. Symptoms are described as more intense and disproportionate to findings on laboratory and physical examination. Extensive overlap exists with signs and symptoms described in chronic fatigue syndrome (see above).

It is associated with irritable bowel syndrome, carpal tunnel syndrome, osteoporosis, Crohn's disease, multiple sclerosis, anemia, seasonal affective disorder, gastroesophageal reflux disease, interstitial cystitis, Sjögren's syndrome, Raynaud's phenomenon, and Morton's neuroma.

Signs and Symptoms

Musculoskeletal pain and stiffness, tension headache, sleep disturbance, fatigue, digestive irritability, emotional alterations and depression, mental changes, coldness, sensations of tingling, poor exercise tolerance, and pain during menses. Symptoms can worsen with exposure to environmental or emotional stress, insomnia, and injury.

Confirmatory Testing

- History—Distribution of pain. Self-ratings of depression, symptom intensity, and life-impact questionnaires.
- Tender Point Screening—Overall tender point score, in addition to eleven or more of the eighteen tender points eliciting abnormal tenderness.
- Blood Studies—Screen for indicators of inflammation and muscle damage as well as underactive thyroid, as the latter has been found to be a common underlying cause of fibromyalgia-type symptoms.

- Specific Laboratory Tests—Tests to rule out other diseases or to confirm suspicions are ordered, based on individual history and presenting signs and symptoms.

Female Health

Part VIII, Section A

Premenstrual Syndrome (PMS)

Premenstrual syndrome is a set of symptoms arising seven to ten days prior to the onset of flow of menses each month. It is most likely caused by a complex interaction of fluctuating levels of hormones. It is associated with lack of essential fatty acids and Vitamin B_6, an underactive thyroid, allergies, impaired carbohydrate metabolism, and an imbalance of intestinal microorganisms.

Signs and Symptoms

Fatigue, transient weight gain, breast enlargement or tenderness, swelling or tingling of the hands and feet, abdominal bloating or cramping, diarrhea and constipation, nausea, vomiting, vertigo, palpitations, headache and backache, pelvic heaviness or pain, altered sex drive, food cravings, acne, emotional alterations and depression, changes in mental function, sleep disturbance, and personality change.

Confirmatory Testing

- History—Symptoms occurring for a minimum of two consecutive months, seven to ten days before the beginning of menses and disappearing by its end.
- Specific Laboratory Tests—Tests to rule out general adaptation syndrome, hormonal imbalance, impaired glucose tolerance, and yeast overgrowth are ordered, depending on the individual history and presenting signs and symptoms.

Anemia

When cells in the kidney detect low oxygen levels in the blood, they signal the production of more red blood cells. This production requires adequate supplies of iron, Vitamin B_{12}, and folate. If these stores are not adequate due to poor intake, absorption, or assimilation of the necessary building blocks, anemia results. Iron-deficiency anemia is the most common type, especially among women and the elderly.

Common causes include: vegetarianism, insufficient stomach acid, bleeding from the digestive tract, malabsorption, heavy menstrual periods, and greater than one past pregnancy.

Signs and Symptoms

Fatigue and shortness of breath with slight exertion, irritability, pale complexion, weakness, drowsiness, vertigo, headache, ringing in the ears, spots before the eyes, loss of sex drive, and scanty menstruation.

Confirmatory Testing

- Blood Studies—Complete blood count, ferritin, vitamin B_{12}, and folate levels.
- Stool Studies—Screen for presence of blood.
- Gastric Acid Analysis—Heidelberg gastric analysis measures the ability of the stomach to secrete acid. Hydrochloric acid challenge uses oral supplementation used to estimate functional stomach acid levels.

Part VIII, Section B

Suboptimal Menopause

Menopause most commonly occurs at fifty-one years of age and marks the completion of menstruation. Many women experience changes in their menstrual cycle during the period leading up to menopause. Some women experience virtually no accompanying symptoms, and others experience severe and debilitating ones.

Signs and Symptoms

Hot flashes, night sweats, palpitations, headaches, difficulty sleeping, emotional alterations, mood swings, mild mental changes, vaginal dryness, bladder and vaginal infections, urinary incontinence, joint pain, fatigue, thinning of hair, acne, dry skin, facial hair, and low sex drive.

Confirmatory Testing

- History—Twelve months since the last menstrual period.
- Physical Examination—Vaginal thinning or dryness, dry skin, thinning of hair, and facial hair.
- Blood Studies—Measure follicle stimulating hormone.

Sleep

Part IX

Insomnia

Your body needs sleep to replenish itself and recover from the stresses of the day. When you don't plan to get enough sleep, you can experience excessive sleepiness during the daytime. Sleep disorders manifest themselves in four different ways: difficulty falling asleep, sleep rhythm disorders, frequent and early awakening, and rebound wakefulness.

Difficulty falling asleep has many causes. Some of the most common are emotional disturbances, but physical problems such as pain, breathing problems, restless legs syndrome, and intake of prescription medication, recreational drugs, alcohol, or stimulants such as coffee, tea, energy drinks, sodas, and chocolate also affect the ability to sleep.

Sleep rhythm disorders occur when people frequently travel across two or more time zones or work irregular hours, failing to sleep at times in line with their natural sleep rhythm.

There are also times when a person wakes frequently or too early and cannot fall back asleep. This is associated with emotional disturbances that may be magnified upon awakening.

Rebound wakefulness occurs when a person stops taking heavy doses of sedative drugs.

Signs and Symptoms

Fatigue, excessive daytime sleepiness, impaired mental and physical function, altered temperature and hormone secretion, a generalized feeling of ill health, irritability, and depression.

Confirmatory Testing

- History—Use of recreational, prescription, or over-the-counter drugs, dietary and beverage intake, degree of psychological stress, shift work, frequent distant travel, and physical activity level.
- Sleep Laboratory Evaluation
- Blood Studies—Measure cortisol, melatonin, and serotonin levels. Screen for presence of low blood sugar.
- Saliva Studies—Measure cortisol and melatonin levels.

Obstructive Sleep Apnea

Sleep apnea is a physical disorder, most commonly experienced by obese people who sleep on their backs. Between periods of snoring, the tissue at the back of the throat relaxes, temporarily blocking airflow to the lungs, and may produce a sensation of choking. This causes a person to both stop breathing and wake throughout the night.

Signs and Symptoms

Restlessness, snoring, recurrent awakening, morning headache, fatigue, excessive daytime sleepiness, and impaired mental and physical function.

Confirmatory Testing

- History—Sleep details obtained from another person or the patient's bed partner.
- Physical Examination—Examination of the nose, mouth, palate, throat, and neck as well as screening for high blood pressure.
- Sleep Evaluation Studies—Measure the frequency and intensity of episodes as well as the oxygen content of the blood.

Limb Movement Disorders

Limb movement disorders are another cause of sleep disturbance. This is characterized by abnormal motions or sensations in the legs that interfere with sleep and may involve abnormalities in dopamine in the brain or be brought on by drug withdrawal, intake of stimulants or medications, chronic kidney or liver impairment, pregnancy, or anemia.

Signs and Symptoms

Interrupted sleep, fatigue, and excessive daytime sleepiness. In restless legs syndrome, specifically, there is a creeping or crawling sensation in the lower extremities upon reclining.

Confirmatory Testing

- History—Sleep details obtained from the patient or patient's bed partner. Information regarding intake of stimulants, medications, drug withdrawal, and pregnancy.
- Sleep Evaluation Studies

- Blood Studies—Screening for anemia, iron deficiency, and liver or kidney dysfunction.

Environmental Health

Part X

Environmental Toxicity

The number and volume of toxic chemicals that are released into our environment daily is staggering. They have a significant impact on our overall state of health and more specifically on our energy levels. Everyday we encounter toxic substances that many people are not even aware of.

Common toxins include: body and home care products, cleaners, soaps, dry cleaning fluids, chlorinated or contaminated water, perfumes, petrochemicals, air and water pollution, clothing, our house and its components, molds and mildews, pollens, plastics, pesticides, herbicides, fungicides, additives, preservatives, vaccinations, over-the-counter and prescription medications, heavy metals (such as mercury, lead, and aluminum), smoking, and recreational drugs.

Environmental toxicity is associated with migraine headaches, autoimmune disorders, depression, ADHD, asthma, chronic fatigue syndrome, fibromyalgia, cancer, multiple chemical sensitivity, Parkinson's disease, and Alzheimer's disease.

Signs and Symptoms

Fatigue and a feeling of sluggishness are among the most common symptoms of toxicity, but the list is too extensive to mention here. If you experience any of these symptoms and fail to find the cause after regular screening, it would be beneficial for you to be assessed for environmental toxicity.

Multiple Chemical Sensitivity

Multiple chemical sensitivity is a chronic disorder characterized by oversensitivity to environmental toxins that are generally well tolerated by others. It is associated with an underactive thyroid gland, autoimmune thyroid disease, impaired metabolism of essential fatty acids and amino acids, as well as deficiencies of magnesium and Vitamin B_6.

Signs and Symptoms

Headaches, depressed mood, hyperactivity, fatigue, skin rash, muscle and joint pain, and inflammation in the nose, sinuses, and throat.

Environmental Toxicity and Multiple Chemical Sensitivity

Confirmatory Testing

- History—Toxic exposure related to community, home, and occupational environments; hobbies and personal habits, including diet and drug intake; development in utero through puberty; and a dental history.

- Specific Laboratory Tests—Tests to rule out other diseases or to confirm suspicions are ordered, based on individual history and on presenting signs and symptoms.

References

1. U.S. Department of Health and Human Services, Centers for Disease Control and Prevention, "Chronic Diseases: The Leading Causes of Death," http://www.cdc.gov/nccdphp/publications/factsheets/ChronicDisease/ (accessed July 7, 2007).

2. National Center for Health Statistics, U.S. Department of Health and Human Services, Centers for Disease Control and Prevention, "Prevalence of Overweight and Obesity among Adults: United States, 2003–2004," http://www.cdc.gov/nchs/products/pubs/pubd/hestats/overweight/ overwght_adult_03.htm (accessed July 27, 2007).

3. M. Tjepkema, "Measured Obesity. Adult Obesity in Canada: Measured Height and Weight," Statistics Canada, Nutrition: Findings from the Canadian Community Health Survey, issue no. 1, http://www.statcan.ca/english/research/82-620MIE/2005001/articles/ adults/aobesity.pdf (accessed October 16, 2007).

4. A. M. Miniño, M. Heron, S. L. Murphy, and K. D. Kochanek, "Deaths: Final Data for 2004," U.S. Department of Health and Human Services, Centers for Disease Control and Prevention, National Center for Health Statistics, http://www.cdc.gov/nchs/products/pubs/pubd/hestats/finaldeaths04/ finaldeaths04.htm (accessed July 27, 2007).

5. Statistics Canada, CANSIM, "Age-standardized Mortality Rates by Selected Causes, by Sex," Table 102-0552, data for 2000–2004, http://www40.statcan.ca/l01/cst01/health30a.htm (accessed July 27, 2007).

6. John Fetto, "Image Is Everything," *American Demographics*, March 1, 2003, http://www.findarticles.com/p/articles/mi_m4021/is_2_25/ai_97818958 (accessed July 27, 2007).

7. National Center for Health Statistics, Department of Health and Human Services, Centers for Disease Control and Prevention, "Health Expenditures,

2004," http://www.cdc.gov/nchs/fastats/hexpense.htm (accessed July 27, 2007).

8. Canadian Institute for Health Information, Statistics Canada, "Health Expenditures, by Type," data for 2000–2004, http://www40.statcan.ca/l01/cst01/health13.htm (accessed January 8, 2007).

9. M. H. Beers, R. S. Porter, T. V. Jones, J. L. Kaplan, and M. Berkwits, eds., *The Merck Manual,* 18th ed. (Whitehouse Station: Merck Research Laboratories, 2006).

10. J. E. Pizzorno and M. T. Murray, eds. *Textbook of Natural Medicine,* 3rd ed. (Philadelphia: Elsevier, 2006).

11. Stephen Covey, *The Seven Habits of Highly Effective People* (New York: Free Press, 2004).

Selected Bibliography

Beers, M., Porter, R, et al. *The Merck Manual.* 18th ed. Whitehouse Station, NJ: Merck Research Laboratories, 2006.

Covey, Stephen. *The Eighth Habit.* New York: Free Press, 2004.

Gladwell, Malcolm. *Blink: The Power of Thinking without Thinking.* New York: Little, Brown and Company, 2005.

Goleman, Daniel. *Emotional Intelligence.* New York: Bantam Dell, 2005.

Heller, Lyra., Katke, Mike. *Health Appraisal Questionnaire,* 1984, revised 2002.

Hill, Napoleon. *John Childers on Think and Grow Rich!* Newport News, VA: Morgan James, 2005.

Pert, Candace. *Molecules of Emotion.* New York: Scribner, 1997.

Pizzorno, J. E., and M. T. Murray, eds. *Textbook of Natural Medicine,* 3rd ed. Philadelphia: Elsevier, 2006.

Rosenberg, Marshall. *Nonviolent Communication.* 2nd ed. USA: PuddleDancer Press, 2003.

Ruiz, Don Miguel. *The Four Agreements.* San Rafael, CA: Amber-Allen, 1997.

Stephen Covey, *The Seven Habits of Highly Effective People.* New York: Free Press, 2004.

Zukav, Gary. *Seat of the Soul.* New York: Simon & Schuster, 1989.

978-0-595-42604-1
0-595-42604-2

Printed in the United States
110039LV00005B/91-150/P